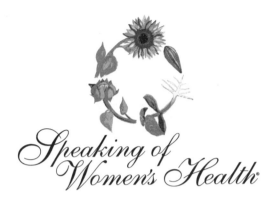

Speaking of Women's Health

SIMPLE PLEDGES:
Building Blocks for Healthy Living

THE BOOK
VOLUME III

D1361154

Introduction

SIMPLE PLEDGES:
Building Blocks for Healthy Living

Congratulations! Because you're reading this book, **SIMPLE PLEDGES:** ***Building Blocks for Healthy Living***, you're taking the first step toward a healthier life. Perfect, because we would like you to join our national campaign **TAKE A PLEDGE FOR BETTER HEALTH™**. This book is designed to make that *simple* for you. Achieving successes through simple pledges are the building blocks that make a strong and beautiful you. Choose one building block, one small positive change in your daily life. What a terrific beginning for your journey to better living!

As you may know, last October, in Wal-Mart stores across the country, Speaking of Women's Health invited women to sign a banner and **TAKE A PLEDGE FOR BETTER HEALTH.** The response was unbelievable! In one weekend, hundreds of thousands of women made a promise to themselves to make one small change. Speaking of Women's Health has now expanded the **TAKE A PLEDGE FOR BETTER HEALTH** program so even more women can share the health!

At Speaking of Women's Health, we believe that you don't have to go to extremes to improve your health, beauty, well-being or personal safety. We *do* believe that just one small change can make a big difference. However long the journey to achieve your goals may seem, it begins with just one small change. Soon, that small change becomes part of your daily routine and a new healthy habit is established. Nothing motivates like success, and when you achieve something, even if it seems small, you should celebrate your success. Not only is being joyful fun (and healthy) *for you*, wait till you see how those around you react! Remember that funny restaurant scene from the movie, *When Harry Met Sally*....when Meg Ryan's character shows a "bit of enthusiasm" and the woman at the next table says, "I'll have what she's having"? What we are all hoping for is happiness and a sense of joy. Feeling better, looking better and being in touch with your spirituality is very achievable and *you* can be the inspiration for those around you by improving your own health, well-being and personal safety.

It all begins with one simple pledge. Ready to get started? Turn the page!

The Staff at
Speaking of Women's Health

A journey of a thousand miles begins with one small step.

This book is designed to provide information about health, not medical advice. Please consult your physician if you have any questions or concerns.

Table of Contents

Letter of Introduction 2

Chapter 1 Healthy Nutrition 6
Awesome Smoothie 15
Delicious Crab Salad 17

Chapter 2 A Physically-Active Life 18
Egg White Omelet 27
White Bean Chili 29

Chapter 3 Healthy Heart 30
Salmon Salad 43
Grilled Kabobs 45

Chapter 4 Healthy Bones 46
Moroccan Couscous Steak Salad 55
Hummus 57

Chapter 5 A Balanced Life 58
Colorful Mashed Potatoes 65
Beef Stew 67

Chapter 6 Hormones
From 15 to Fabulous! 68
Chicken Soup 79
Vi's Sunday Greens 81

Chapter 7 Beauty and Healthy Skin 82
Traditional Gazpacho 95
Chalupa 97

Chapter 8 Trust Your Gut 98
Beef & Broccoli with Ginger 109
Apple & Apricot Stuffed Pork Chops 111

Chapter 9 Aging Gracefully 112
Rolled Chicken 121
Peppermint Patty Cheesecake 123

Chapter 10 Personal and
Family Safety 124
Oats & Honey Bread 139
Party Pizzas 141

Index 142

The nutritional analysis provided is not intended for medical nutrition therapy. If you are following a strict diet for medical or dietary reasons, consult first with a physician or dietician before planning your meals.

OUR HOSPITAL PARTNERS*

*S*peaking of Women's Health is proud to partner with these hospitals to provide the latest, most up-to-date educational resources and information. At Speaking of Women's Health, our mission is to "educate women to make informed decisions about their health, well-being and personal safety". We have partnered with these health care institutions because we feel they have shared goals and a common vision with us.

Tri Health Women's Health: Bethesda North and Good Samaritan	Cincinnati, OH
Mercy Health Partners	Cincinnati, OH
The Cleveland Clinic	Cleveland, OH
St. Vincent Women's Hospital	Indianapolis, IN
Shawnee Mission Medical Center	Kansas City
Boone Hospital Center	Columbia, MO
Baptist Health	Jacksonville, FL
King's Daughters Hospital and Health Services	Madison, IN
St. Anthony's Medical Center	Merrillville, IN
The Cleveland Clinic Florida	Miami, FL
Washington Regional Medical Center	Northwest, AR
Orlando Regional Hospital	Orlando, FL
Strong Health	Rochester, NY
Miami Valley Hospital	Dayton, OH
The Women's Pavilion at St. Mark's Hospital	Salt Lake City, UT
Sharp Health Care System	San Diego, CA
Manatee Memorial Hospital & Health System	Sarasota, FL
H. Lee Moffitt Cancer Center and Research Institute	Tampa Bay, FL
Covenant Health System	Waterloo, IA
Sara Lee Center for Women's Health at Forsyth Medical Center	Winston-Salem, NC

*as of this printing

A special thanks to Shawnee Mission Medical Center in Kansas City for providing nutritional analysis for the recipes listed in SIMPLE PLEDGES: Building Blocks for Healthy Living.

Shawnee Mission Medical Center is home of the Center for Women's Health and recognized as one of the nation's 10 best hospitals for women by *Self* magazine. The hospital prides itself on meeting the unique needs of women throughout their lifespan. Our goal is to empower women with the knowledge they need to become active participants in their health care and to promote good health for life.

Chapter 1
Healthy Nutrition

"Do you eat to live or live to eat? With knowledge and a zest for life, you don't have to choose."

Anonymous

A simple pledge...

for a nutritious diet begins with the delight of adding a few brightly colored fruits and vegetables to your diet each week. This chapter will give you lots of suggestions for adding delicious and nutritious foods that will be your building blocks for healthy living.

Every living being requires nourishment to grow and survive. Even machines require fuel to run. The human body is certainly no exception.

Food not only fuels our bodies, it also awakens our senses. Nature has given us the best of everything when it comes to food. We now know that the most beautifully-colored foods are also the most nutritious. And, when used in recipes, combining foods can make a beautiful presentation, have intoxicating aromas, fill our mouths with wonderful textures and flavors and create memories. So, food is clearly more than *just* fuel. Food also provides energy. That energy is what we commonly call calories. Let's explore the relationships and how to make it all work *for* us.

Nutrition experts have long understood the connection between food and energy. More recently, athletes have been very influential in communicating the positive messages about healthy eating. Even the creators of Popeye knew that spinach was a great source for energy and strength, and, in fact, upon the cartoon's debut in 1929, spinach became one of the most popular children's foods. The U.S. Government has established new dietary guidelines which we will discuss in this chapter.

Control Calorie Intake To Manage Body Weight

It's not news to most of us that American adults and children are in the middle of an obesity epidemic. The government's advisors say that calorie intake and physical activity go hand-in-hand to control body weight. To maintain a healthy body weight, calories consumed should be equal to or less than calories expended.

The simplest way to reduce calories is to watch portion sizes, and reduce your intake of added sugars and alcohol...and balance this with exercise. See Chapter 2 for more information and helpful hints on exercise.

Choose Fats Wisely For Good Health

Some fats are healthier for you than others – distinguishing between the two may be tricky. The nutrition experts at Cleveland Clinic Foundation describe the two basic types of fats:

Hydrogenated (Trans) Fats – found in processed foods, margarines and fried foods. These should be minimized.

Healthy Fats like the Omega-3 fats are – found in some fish, nuts, avocados, flaxseed. Omega-6 fats are found in low-fat dairy and lean proteins. These essential fats can be eaten more frequently.

Total fat intake for healthy adults should be less than 30% of calories consumed, with saturated fats below 10% of calories, and trans fats below 1% of calories. Nutritionists suggest keeping saturated fats low by limiting animal fats. Choose lean meats and low or non-fat varieties of cheese, milk, yogurt and other dairy products. To keep trans fats down, limit all foods prepared with partially hydrogenated vegetable oils.

Choose Carbohydrates Wisely For Good Health

When dieting, be careful not to totally eliminate carbs. Limiting carbs may also limit energy. The government guidelines view carbohydrates as an important part of a healthy diet and the major energy source in most diets.

Carbohydrates are one of three "macronutrients" in our diets that provide calories. The other two are protein and fat. Carbohydrates provide most of the energy needed in our daily lives, both for normal body functions such as heartbeat, breathing and digestion, as well as for physical activities such as walking and running.

In the past few years, more and more nutrition experts recommend incorporating complex carbs into your diet, and cutting down on simple carbs. Why?

Simple carbohydrates are digested quickly. Many simple carbohydrates contain refined sugars and few essential vitamins and minerals. Most of the simple carbs we consume should come from fruits and milk or yogurt.

Complex carbohydrates take longer to digest and are usually packed with healthy essentials such as fiber, vitamins and minerals. The bulk of the carbs we consume should be complex. Samples of complex carbohydrates include whole or multi-grained breads, cereals and pasta; brown rice; peas; beans and lentils.

Increase Daily Intake Of Fruits And Vegetables, Whole Grains And Reduced-Fat Milk And Milk Products

Your Mom always told you to eat your veggies! And, **the good news is**…she was right. Healthy adults should strive for 5 servings of fruits and vegetables each day, as a minimum. A single serving may not be as much as you think. If you choose a salad for lunch, that may count for as many as 3 servings of veggies. Why? Because a serving is ½ cup. Add an apple for a snack and some berries on your morning cereal and you've got 5 locked up.

Choose And Prepare Foods That Are Low In Salt

According to the FDA (Food and Drug Administration), reducing salt intake is one way to lower blood pressure – which is important in preventing stroke, heart disease and kidney failure. To find out if the foods you eat are high in salt, check the nutrition label for sodium. Strive for less than 2,300 milligrams of sodium per day.

One easy way to reduce sodium is to reach for herbs, pepper or garlic powder instead of the salt shaker. Many favorite foods are now available in low-sodium or no-salt options. Additionally, health-conscious frozen meals are also now available in low-sodium, low-fat varieties, complete with whole grains.

One of the best nutrition tips we've heard comes from Speaking of Women's Health national speaker and author, Victoria Moran. Moran encourages women to simply "choose the best of what's available". This means that wherever you are, make the best choice from what is offered, and limit portion sizes. If you absolutely cannot resist temptation and must splurge on something sinfully delicious…go ahead! But, please, savor each and every bite and enjoy it to its fullest! If you make healthy choices 90% of the time…you're doing great! There's nothing wrong with an occasional reward that may not be great for your body, but may be great for your soul!

Building Blocks...
for Healthy Nutrition

According to the U.S. Government guidelines, choose foods from the 6 food groups, in the recommended amounts:

Proteins . . . . 2 to 3 servings daily
Dairy. . . . . 2 to 3 servings daily
Carbohydrates. . . . . 6 to 11 servings daily
Fruits . . . . 2 to 4 servings daily
Vegetables. . . . . 3 to 5 servings daily
Fats, oils & sweets. . . . . Use sparingly

See page 13 for serving sizes.

Consider these healthy carbohydrate recommendations:
- ✔ Multi-grain or whole-wheat bread
- ✔ Whole-grain cereals
- ✔ Low or non-fat dairy including milk, yogurt and cheeses
- ✔ Brown rice, whole grain orzo
- ✔ Fresh fruits, with skin on
- ✔ Vegetables

Consider these healthy proteins:
- ✔ Lean meats
- ✔ Nuts
- ✔ Fish
- ✔ Poultry
- ✔ Eggs or egg whites

Consider these "good" fat sources:
- ✔ Fish (Omega-3s)
- ✔ Nuts
- ✔ Avocados
- ✔ Olive, Canola oils
- ✔ Low-fat dairy (Omega-6s)

Here are some of nature's most health-full foods, and suggested ways to add them into your daily food choices:

Almonds – Nuts are a great source of protein, and almonds are one of the best. Keep 10-15 handy to snack on throughout the day.

Flaxseed – Eat ground flax, along with other nuts and seeds, for a boost of protein, good fats and other nutrients. Flax is good for your heart, hair, nails, eyes and skin, and toss it into the foods of the men in your life to improve prostate health.

Kiwi – A recent study suggests that bite for bite, kiwifruit contains more essential nutrients than 32 of the most popular fruits, making it one of the most "nutrient dense" fruits in the world. Kiwifruit is also a good source of magnesium, is sodium-free and is a low-fat source of Vitamin E.

Mango – Loaded with Vitamins A, B, C, carotenoids (helps ward off colds), fiber, calcium, iron and potassium. WOW!

Soy – Two good sources of soy protein include soy milk, a delicious alternative for those who are lactose intolerant; and, edamame (green soybeans in a pod) that come fresh or frozen. Edamame are low in carbs and a great protein source.

Oats – The high fiber content helps remove cholesterol from the digestive system.

Peppermint – A rich source of manganese and Vitamins A & C, peppermint oils found in leaves have been shown to soothe muscle spasms from irritable bowel syndrome and have antioxidant effects. Also, its aroma aids in relaxation and revitalization. (If you suffer from GERD, you may want to avoid peppermint. See page 100.)

Tea – A cup of good health! Tea contains polyphenols that act like antioxidants. Green and white teas are the best. Tea may help control cholesterol, reduce tooth decay, and prevent stroke, heart disease and intestinal cancers.

One key ingredient to look for in all foods you consume is color! Strive to incorporate color into all of your food choices and mix colors together for a bright and lively meal. If you think of it very simply – color equals nutrition…you can't go wrong. Now, of course, not all color is from a natural source…but, as Victoria Moran says… "Pretty Groceries Make Pretty People!" Challenge yourself to serve meals bursting with natural color and goodness. Look for dark green leafy vegetables, rich red beets, apricot colored mangoes, minty green kiwi, bright beautiful salmon, berries of all colors…got the picture?

Finally, our bodies cannot survive without water! Think of water as nature's perfect nutrient…it's found nearly everywhere, it's often free, and it contains no calories…so, drink to your health!

Simple Pledges...
for Healthy "On-The-Go" Snacking

Many healthy snacks and meal replacements are available. Be sure to check the label for recommended serving sizes.

I pledge to: ☑

❏ Pack a yogurt for a mid-morning snack.

❏ Choose ½ cup trail mix for an afternoon snack or as a treat before bedtime.

❏ Prepare a fruit smoothie for breakfast. (See recipe page 15.)

❏ Keep carrot sticks and cut celery in the refrigerator or, take with me to work.

❏ Keep a delicious and nutritious meal replacement bar or drink on hand for busy days.

Keep Your Body Hydrated!
Here are some simple tips to help keep your body hydrated...

✔ Fill a water bottle in the morning and sip on it throughout the day. Refill as needed.

✔ Got a craving or thinking about a snack? STOP! Drink 8 ounces of water and wait 10 minutes. If you're still hungry...then eat a healthy snack.

✔ Drink a glass of water about 15 minutes before each meal. This helps your body digest food, and helps you feel more full, so it will be easier to watch portion sizes.

TAKE A PLEDGE FOR BETTER HEALTH at www.speakingofwomenshealth.com

Speaking Of Portion Sizes...How Much Is Enough?

Generally speaking, Americans eat too much! A serving size or portion is not defined by the amount that will fit onto a plate! And, when reading food labels, don't be fooled...look at the number of servings per container...it is often more than you think. For example, if one serving has 160 calories, that's not so bad! BUT...if there are 3 servings per container, and you consume the entire container...that 160 calories jumps to 480! Beware!

A great way to gauge correct portion sizes is to make sure it fits into the palm of your hand. Or, is it roughly the size of a deck of cards? If each serving of food on your plate is smaller than a deck of cards, then you're on the right track.

What Is A Serving Size?

Fruits	½ cup chopped fruit or 1 medium piece of fruit, ¾ cup juice or ¾ ounce of dried fruit (this is about one handful).
Veggies	1 cup raw green leaves or ½ cup cooked or raw veggies or ¾ cup of juice.
Grains	1 cup cereal or 1 slice whole wheat bread, ½ cup cooked rice or grain or ½ cup cooked pasta.
Fish, meat, poultry or legumes	1 serving (3 oz.) cooked fish, beef or other meat or ½ cup legumes.
Fat	1 teaspoon butter, oil or peanut butter, 1 tablespoon regular salad dressing or ½ ounce nuts.
Dairy	1 cup fat-free or 1% milk, 1 cup fat-free or low-fat yogurt or 1 ounce low-fat cheese.

For all that we do know about nutrition, there is still much that we have yet to learn. The fact is, the best PLEDGE FOR BETTER HEALTH that you can make is very simple...eat a variety of foods that are colorful and that you enjoy, following the guidelines discussed in this chapter. Cook from scratch when possible, and when it's not...choose the best from what's available. If this is a frozen meal, seek low sodium and proper portion control. If "what's available" is a restaurant, choose your foods wisely and again, watch portion sizes.

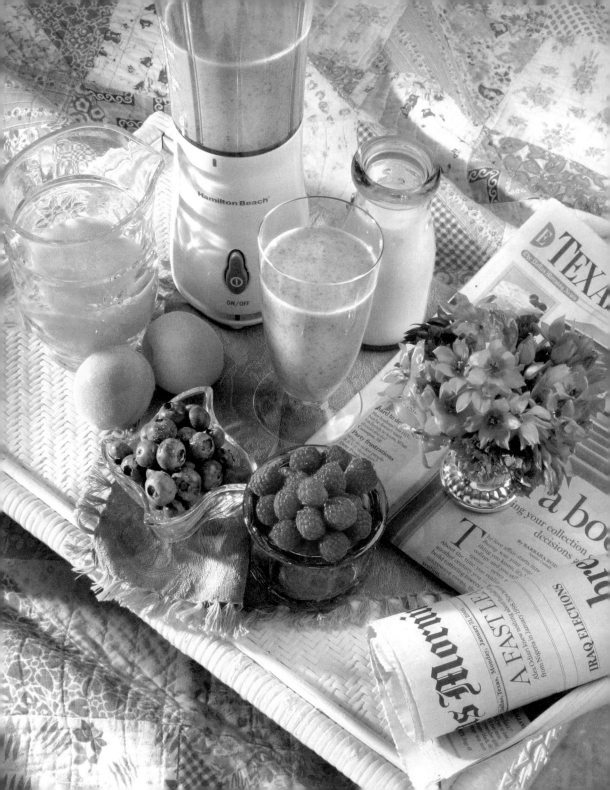

Awesome Smoothies

Thanks to Florence Henderson
National Honorary Chair, Speaking of Women's Health

A smoothie is a nutritious treat for breakfast, or anytime you want a pick-me-up! Have fun experimenting with different flavors by including your favorite berries and seasonal fruits.

INGREDIENTS

2 Tbsp.	ground flaxseed
1	banana
1 cup	low-fat or fat-free fruit yogurt
1½ cups	frozen blueberries or strawberries *(peaches, mangoes, raspberries)*
1 cup	low-fat soy milk

PREPARATION

• Place all ingredients in blender and process until desired texture.

A smoothie is a great way to add additional vitamins and nutrients into your diet. Consider adding a protein powder, fiber supplement, wheat germ, or other herbal supplements in powder form, just as this recipe suggests ground flaxseed. Remember what Mary Poppins said, "Just a spoonful of sugar..."? Well, in this case, it's a spoonful of smoothie! Enjoy!

NUTRITIONAL ANALYSIS
Servings per recipe: 2
Each serving contains approximately:
113 calories
5 g. protein
19 g. carbohydrates
3 g. fat (No saturated fat!)
8 mg. calcium

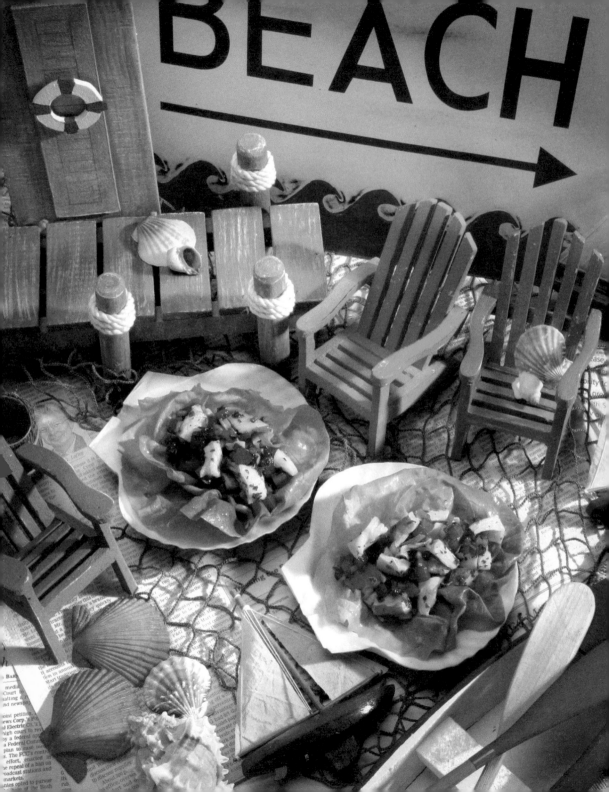

Delicious Crab Salad

Thanks to Isaac Benchimol
Retail Promotion Manager, Wal-Mart Team, Pfizer, Inc.

This is a delicious and healthy salad that we like to eat wrapped in lettuce! Lettuce wraps are a healthy new trend. You can use lettuce to wrap any salad or rice dish...or, for a "lite" change, substitute lettuce for bread and wrap your favorite sandwich!

INGREDIENTS

Salad

8 oz.	crabmeat *(real or imitation)*
½	red bell pepper
½	yellow or orange bell pepper
6	scallions, white and green parts
1	clove garlic, minced *(optional)*
1	small carrot
5-6	leaves Romaine lettuce
3	leaves radicchio
4	large leaves, Bibb lettuce
	A fist-size bunch fresh Italian parsley *(stems removed)*

Vinaigrette Dressing

6 Tbsp.	vegetable or olive oil
2½ to 3 Tbsp.	balsamic vinegar

PREPARATION

Salad

- Finely chop all the ingredients, except Bibb lettuce and place them into a large bowl.

Vinaigrette Dressing

- In a small bowl, whisk together the ingredients.
- Pour enough dressing on the salad to moisten.
- Toss well, serve immediately, and enjoy!

ASSEMBLY: WRAP & ROLL

- Spoon salad into the Bibb lettuce leaves. Use 2 leaves per wrap.

NUTRITIONAL ANALYSIS
Servings per recipe: 2
Each serving contains approximately:
206 calories
13 g. protein
16 g. carbohydrates
10 g. fat (1 g. saturated fat)

Chapter 2
A Physically-Active Life

"Only those who have the patience to do simple things perfectly ever acquire the skill to do difficult things easily."

Unknown

A simple pledge...

*for a physically-active lifestyle
begins with finding an activity that
brings you joy and finding
someone to share it with.*

If someone told you that there was a "magic pill" that could improve your heart health, help you maintain or lose weight, build strong bones to prevent osteoporosis, keep your mind sharp, improve your sexual life, decrease your chance of cancers, and…improve your overall sense of well-being…would you jump at the chance to get it? YES? Well, today is your lucky day…because, that "magic pill" is physical activity! And, it's available to you free of charge and in many convenient forms.

At Speaking of Women's Health, we often substitute the words "pleasurable physical activity" for "exercise". The concept of exercise and the joy of pleasurable physical activity are certainly not mutually exclusive. Consider this survey: Researchers at the University of Arkansas report that women aged 50 and over, who gardened on a regular basis, had higher bone density readings than those whose activity was what we tend to think of as "exercise". This makes sense when you think of all of the bending, stretching, pulling, pushing and carrying that is associated with gardening. The added bonus is that gardening is pleasant and may also lower stress! Skincare experts remind us to always protect with sunscreen of at least SPF (sun protection factor) 15, and stay hydrated when working outdoors.

*For all
that we know
about the benefits
of physical
activity, many
women
(roughly 60%)
still do not engage
in activity!
If you're one of
them...GET
MOVING!*

So, whether it's gardening, team sports, tennis, golf, weight-bearing exercise at the gym, yoga or simply walking with a friend...here are some of the health benefits that come from engaging in pleasurable activities.

The key is, if you engage in 30 minutes of activity most days, you could:

✔ Lower your blood pressure

✔ Improve your sleep

✔ Increase oxygen to the brain and improve memory and mental alertness

✔ Make your bones stronger and improve your posture

✔ Burn stored body fat to help you lose weight

✔ Increase energy

✔ Increase your metabolism to convert more calories to energy and less to stored fat

✔ Protect your body from injury and disease

✔ Slow the aging process

✔ Look better with a toned body and healthy skin

✔ Boost self-confidence

With all of these benefits, why not **TAKE A PLEDGE FOR BETTER HEALTH** for 30 minutes of pleasurable physical activity every day.

Building Blocks...
for "Pleasurable Activity"

Exercise doesn't have to be tedious. It can be one of your most pleasurable activities. Let's look at other types of exercise or activity.

Weight-Bearing Activity

First, there's *weight-bearing* exercise. The key to weight-bearing exercise is that your body must bear its own weight. Bicycling is a great exercise, but the bike is bearing your weight, so it's not weight-bearing – the same with swimming because the water is bearing your weight. Think walking, using hand weights, carrying groceries, dancing, bowling, golfing (carry your own bag) and even gardening. If you belong to a gym, use the machines to work all major muscle groups – arms, chest, back, stomach, hips and legs. Weight-bearing exercise is important to improve muscle strength and build bones.

Aerobic Activity

Then there's *aerobic*...this is any exercise that uses large muscle groups in a continuous, rhythmic fashion for a sustained amount of time to get the heart and lungs working and pumping. Aerobic exercise includes bicycling, swimming, jogging or brisk walking, dancing, playing volleyball, tennis, racquetball, soccer, softball or basketball, skating. Aerobic exercise helps strengthen your heart muscles to keep them working effectively.

Stretching Activity

Stretching is essential for maintaining muscle health and increased flexibility. Many women complain of chronic back pain...if you're one of them...then begin and end each day with gentle stretching to encourage your back muscles to loosen up. Yoga is a great activity that focuses on balance, breathing, strength building and flexibility. It combines deep breathing, relaxation and mindful focus while you stretch and balance in simple, easy postures. Look for beginner's videos to follow, or seek out a class in your neighborhood or near your work.

Shoe Tips!

Good shoes, appropriate for the sport or activity, can make a world of difference in the results. Ill-fitting shoes can cause foot, leg, knee and hip pain, especially if they're worn out or don't have the kind of support you need for your body type or the particular activity you're doing.

✔ *Try on shoes after a workout at the end of the day, when your feet are the largest.*

✔ *Wear the same socks you'll be wearing during the activity.*

✔ *Forget about a "break in" period. If they don't fit in the store or are uncomfortable... keep looking.*

✔ *The heel should fit firmly with no slipping and you should be able to wiggle all of your toes.*

Consider keeping a pair of walking shoes and socks in your car so you can take advantage of opportunities that arise for walking and activity.

Dress For Success!

Comfort is very important for activity. Choose light-weight clothing that breathes and allows moisture to evaporate or materials that actually wick away moisture from your skin. Affordable exercise clothing can be found almost anywhere, and today's styles are even fashionable enough to wear outside of the gym. Be sure your clothing does not restrict movement or cause discomfort. Also, wear a supportive bra that fits properly to relieve breast discomfort.

Wearing The Wrong Bra Size?

Tired of tugging, fidgeting and strategically lifting one arm to "adjust" your bra strap? You're not alone. In a recent survey, 86% of the women surveyed thought they were wearing the right bra size, when in truth, more than 70% of these women were actually wearing the wrong size. A bra that doesn't fit properly can cause poor posture, shoulder strain, pinching and binding. And let's face it...it's just UNCOMFORTABLE!

How To Choose A Proper Fit

For correct band length, measure directly under the breasts and add 5 inches. **For correct cup size,** pull a tape measure up under the arms and measure at the top of the chest wall. For each inch over the band size, add one cup size (1" = A, 2" = B, and so on). Half sizes are now available for a more customized fit.

Most women have one breast that is larger than the other. Always fit the cup size to the fuller breast first. Every woman should reassess her bra size yearly, especially after a major life change, such as having a baby, weight gain or loss of more than 10 pounds or taking on a new exercise regimen.

Be Smart About How You Add Activity

Even with moderate activity, dehydration from lack of water intake is a major cause of fatigue, poor performance, decreased coordination and muscle cramping. Proper hydration is extremely important before, during and after exercise. The longer and more intensely you work out, the more you'll need to drink.

✔ Drink 2 glasses of fluid a few hours before exercise.

✔ Drink every 15 minutes during exercise.

✔ Keep drinks cooler than air temperature and close at hand. Consider adding a few lemon slices or mint leaves to your water to make it taste fresh.

✔ If you exercise more than 60 minutes, you may benefit from a sports drink containing carbohydrates.

TAKE A PLEDGE FOR BETTER HEALTH

Despite the many benefits of physical activity, many women tell us that they just cannot commit to making it happen. It may be that you feel guilty taking time out of the family's hectic schedule for yourself. As women, we tend to put ourselves last…if this is what you do, your building blocks will tumble. The stronger you are, both mentally and physically, the better able you'll be to take care of the others in your life who depend on you. Remember, you're not alone…in fact; you might invite a group of other women in similar situations to either exercise together, or take turns watching the kids while you exercise. For every challenge, there is a solution. Get your creative juices flowing and figure out a simple way to make it happen. You'll be rewarded with a healthier, more toned body and a sharper mind. And, most importantly…a sense of relaxation!

Single sports and team sports are great physical activities that not only burn calories and help build bone mass, they're also great stress reducers and a wonderful way to build friendships and team-thinking. Think about racquetball, tennis, golf, soccer, baseball, volleyball, badminton played in the backyard…call some friends and have some fun!

Simple Pledges...
for a Physically-Active Lifestyle

I pledge to: ☑

❏ Set the alarm early on Monday morning and start off the work week with a 30-minute walk before work.

❏ Meet my child's bus and walk home…the long way! If we take turns carrying the backpack, we will both build strong bones!

❏ Invite other parents to join me in circling the soccer field for 30 minutes or walking the halls at school during basketball practice. I will keep some free weights in my desk and car so I can take advantage of downtime to build arm strength.

❏ Enjoy a yoga video or dvd or, join a class at the Y or yoga studio.

❏ Shorten my lunch and take a walk with co-workers. Have a meeting? Ask the participant to go for a walk and talk, instead of sitting at a desk or table…then send a quick e-mail to recap the discussion and next steps.

❏ Make a date night with my spouse and go dancing!

❏ Look for ways to incorporate weight-bearing exercise into my housecleaning routine… carrying laundry up and down stairs, bringing groceries into the house, bending to load and unload the dishwasher.

TAKE A PLEDGE FOR BETTER HEALTH at www.speakingofwomenshealth.com

Simple Pledges...
for a Physically-Active Lifestyle

I pledge to: ☑

❑ Make errand day, activity day! Park in one central location and walk to the drycleaner, video store and library.

❑ After dinner, ask the kids to clean up while my spouse and I, or neighbor, go for a walk.

❑ Start my morning off with 10 minutes of gentle stretching to energize and wake up my body. (This is a great way to end the day, also!)

❑ Take a walk after my religious services to reflect on the day's messages.

❑ Enjoy my favorite TV program, the guilt-free way. I will do some leg lifts and stretching during the commercial breaks.

❑ Put on my walking shoes and go for it...get some shopping done! I will challenge myself to move throughout the store and walk each aisle for added activity.

TAKE A PLEDGE FOR BETTER HEALTH at www.speakingofwomenshealth.com

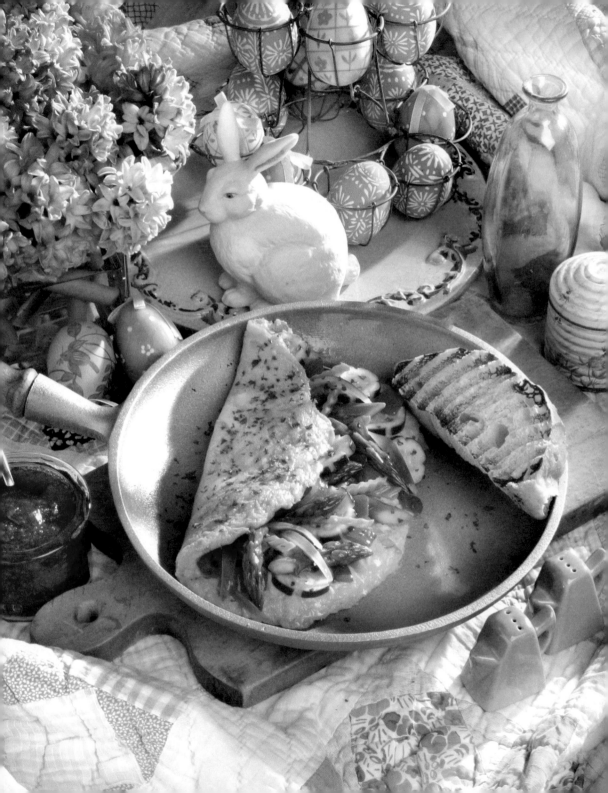

Egg White Omelet

Thanks to Robert Lack
Buyer, Dry Grocery, Wal-Mart

A great and healthy way to start your day is with a delicious, veggie-filled egg white omelet. Substitute your favorite seasonal vegetables and try different low-fat cheeses for flavor…you can't go wrong!

INGREDIENTS

8   egg whites, 4 per omelet
    cooking spray

    tons of veggies – onions, mushrooms, tomatoes, broccoli, asparagus, shallots, garlic

    herbs – fresh basil, parsley, rosemary, salt & pepper to taste

    low-fat or fat-free cheese, if desired

    You can also use cholesterol-free egg substitute in place of egg whites. Cook according to directions.

PREPARATION

• Lightly sauté veggies in olive oil.

• Coat omelet pan with cooking spray and heat.

• Whisk egg whites until frothy and pour into hot pan.

• Loosen the sides of the omelet — when the whites have partially firmed, carefully turn it over and cook the other side.

• Place veggies and cheese, if desired, in the center of the omelet.

• Fold the omelet over the vegetables. Garnish with additional herbs and cheese.

NUTRITIONAL ANALYSIS
Servings: 2
Each serving contains approximately:
134 calories
12 g. protein
1 g. carbohydrates
7 g. fat (2 g. saturated fat)
38 mg. calcium

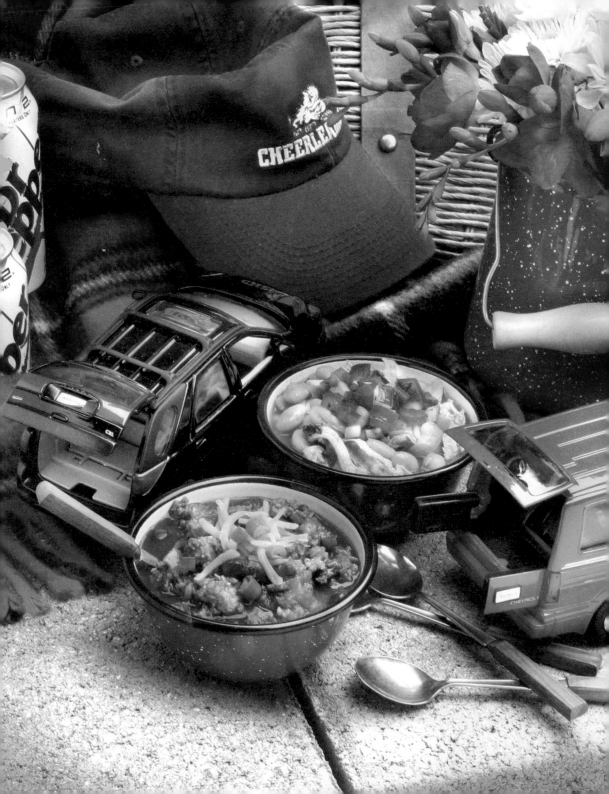

White Bean Chili

Thanks to Katie Taylor
Chief Customer Officer, Sara Lee Branded Apparel (Hanes)

Try this healthy and great-tasting twist on your favorite chili recipe. White Bean Chili is full of calcium and healthy nutrients, and a good source of complex carbs.

INGREDIENTS

1½ lbs.	skinless chicken breasts
4 - 14 oz. cans	reduced sodium chicken broth
3 - 14 oz. cans	white northern beans
1 - 14 oz. can	white kidney beans
2 heaping tsp.	cumin
2 heaping tsp.	oregano
2 tsp.	chili powder
1 tsp.	cayenne pepper
	couple of dashes of your favorite hot sauce
2 Tbsp.	chopped garlic
2 cups	chopped onions
2 Tbsp.	olive oil
1 - 4 oz. can	chopped green chilies
	salt and pepper to taste

PREPARATION

- Season chicken breasts with salt and pepper. Poach in 2 cans chicken broth for approximately 15 minutes depending on size. Chicken should be fully cooked, not pink in middle. Keep at a very low simmer, otherwise chicken will be tough.

- While chicken is poaching, combine chicken broth, white northern beans, white kidney beans, cumin, oregano, chili powder, cayenne pepper, and hot sauce in a 6-quart stock pot.

- Sauté garlic and onions in olive oil until tender.

- Add green chilies and sauté 2 more minutes. Add to other ingredients.

- When chicken is poached, let cool and cut or tear into bite-sized pieces.

- Add chicken to chicken stock mixture.

- Cook for at least one hour and serve.

NUTRITIONAL ANALYSIS
Servings per recipe: 6
Each serving contains approximately:
275 calories
33 g. protein
10 g. carbohydrates
10 g. fat (2 g. saturated fat)
29 mg. calcium

Chapter 3
Healthy Heart

"I am beginning to learn that it is the
sweet, simple things of life which are the real
ones after all."

Laura Ingalls Wilder

A simple pledge...

*for a healthy heart begins
with understanding how your
heart can make you happy, strong
and beautiful every day.*

It's not by accident that "heart" has become synonymous with terms meaning the center, core, soul or most-vital ingredient. The "heart" of the home is the family, the "heart" of the matter is the key point, the "heart" is the symbol for love and a "beating heart" is the symbol of life. In fact, when we "make a pledge", even as children, we cross our hearts and when we say the Pledge of Allegiance, we place our hand over our hearts. So clearly, we need to protect something so precious and vital to our very existence!

The heart's job is simple... it moves blood!

Blood nourishes all of the organs with oxygen. So, if there's not enough pumping, the organs may not receive enough oxygen. Too much causes the heart muscles to fatigue, which means they don't work properly.

To better understand your heart, think of it as a house. Inside, it consists of four rooms, or chambers, that hold the blood and nourish it with oxygen; four doors, or valves that open to allow blood flow throughout; and, of course, hallways or vessels, that carry the blood into and out of the house.

The plumbing, or vessels in the heart, delivers fresh blood from the aorta to supply the walls of the heart with blood. The walls of the heart are very important muscles which squeeze and relax so the heart can push the blood out. The walls of the heart are made of muscle. When the walls squeeze (contract) they push the blood out to the body. When the walls relax, they allow the heart to fill with blood again. This cycle happens about 70 times per minute. To do so, the muscles of the heart must get enough blood. Heart attacks happen when the blood supply to the muscles of the heart is blocked.

Like any house, your heart also consists of an electrical system. When you walk into your house, you switch on a light. When you flip the switch, it sends an electrical impulse throughout the room to turn on the lights. Each time the sinus node in your heart fires, it sends an electrical impulse throughout the heart, causing it to beat. The sinus node is what is known as your heart's pacemaker. If it fires too much, you may have a rapid heart rhythm, too little firing causes a slow rhythm.

Sudden cardiac arrest, or **SCA**, is the sudden, abrupt loss of heart function caused by an interruption in the heart's electrical system, occurring in a person who may or may not have been diagnosed with heart disease.

As we've said, a heart attack occurs when the path becomes blocked and blood cannot reach the heart. A stroke, or "brain attack", occurs when the blood supply to the brain is cut off.

A Healthy Heart

The heart is a complex organ, yet keeping it healthy is relatively simple. **The good news is** that what's good for the heart is also healthy for the rest of your body. A healthy, low-fat diet helps keep fatty substances (caused by cholesterol) from building up in your "pipes" or arteries. These fatty substances, known as plaque, may block the pathway of blood into and out of the heart and throughout the body.

Some causes of heart disease are not controllable, except through awareness. Factors such as age, family history and race all contribute to our heart's health. It is helpful to know your family history so that you can alter your personal lifestyle to help compensate. Understanding your risk factors for heart disease or stroke can save your life.

Let's Take A Closer Look

Heart attack and stroke are not only a concern for men. Heart attack, stroke and other cardiovascular diseases are also devastating to women. In fact, coronary heart disease, which causes heart attack, is the leading cause of death for American women. Many women believe that cancer is more of a threat, but they're wrong. Nearly twice as many women in the United States die of heart disease and stroke as from all forms of cancer, including breast cancer. **The good news is** that heart disease and stroke can be minimized through a healthy lifestyle.

The American Heart Association has identified several factors that increase the risk of heart disease and stroke. The more risk factors a woman has, the greater her risk of a heart attack or stroke. While you can't control some risk factors, others can be controlled through a modified lifestyle.

Exercise, or physical activity, is essential to keep your muscles strong and to generate oxygen throughout the body. Physical activity also helps keep the arteries free of plaque, and helps your body convert food into energy. Exercise also helps reduce unhealthy stress.

Simple Pledges for a Heart Healthy Diet

TAKE A PLEDGE today to eat a diet low in fat and cholesterol and to keep your "pipes" clear of fatty buildup.

✔ **Get your Cs...** *Vitamin C, that is. These rich antioxidants help rid your bloodstream of free radicals, which can contribute to heart disease.*

✔ **Eat Fish...** *A healthy heart needs Omega-3 fatty acids, found in some fish – anchovies, bluefish, herring, salmon, sardines, canned light tuna. Omega-3s are also found in canola oil and flaxseed.*

✔ **Magnificent magnesium...** *Recent studies suggest that magnesium may help coordinate the activity of the heart muscle, as well as the functioning of the nerves that initiate the heartbeat. It also helps keep coronary arteries from spasming, an action that can cause the intense chest pain known as angina. Magnesium is found in cereals, root vegetables, seafood, legumes, whole grains, nuts and seeds.*

✔ **Potent potassium...** *Potassium is essential to help maintain the normal function of the heart and nervous system. Good sources include fresh fruit (bananas), dried fruit, legumes, potatoes, tomatoes, seafood and milk.*

What Are The Risk Factors For Heart Disease And Stroke That You Can't Control?

Increasing age. As women grow older, their risk of heart disease and stroke increases, particularly after menopause.

Sex *(Gender)*. Men have a greater risk of heart attack than do women, and their attacks often occur at a younger age. However, more women die from first-time heart attacks than do men. Each year about 40,000 more women than men have strokes, and more than 60% of total stroke deaths occur in women.

Heredity *(family history)*. Both women and men are more likely to develop heart disease or stroke if a close blood relative has had either. Race is also a factor. Women of color have a greater risk of heart disease and stroke than white women. Compared to Caucasians, both African-American men and women are more likely to die of stroke.

Previous heart attack or stroke or TIA. Women who've had a heart attack are at higher risk of having a second heart attack. 14% of those who survive a first stroke or heart attack will have another within one year. A transient ischemic attack (TIA or "mini-stroke") also is a risk factor and predictor of stroke.

What Risk Factors Can Be Modified, Treated Or Controlled By Focusing On Lifestyle Habits And Taking Medicine, If Needed?

Tobacco smoke. Smoking is the single most preventable cause of death in the United States. Smoking is a major cause of coronary artery disease (heart attack) among women. Women who smoke also have an increased risk for stroke. Exposure to second-hand smoke at work or at home, also increases the risk, even for nonsmokers.

Women who smoke and use birth control pills have a higher risk of heart attack and stroke than nonsmokers using birth control pills.

High blood cholesterol. High blood cholesterol is a major risk factor for heart disease and also increases the risk of stroke. Studies show that a woman's cholesterol is higher than a man's from age 45 on. High levels of **LDL** (low-density lipoprotein) cholesterol (the "bad" cholesterol – think "L" for lousy) **raise the risk** of heart disease and heart attack. High levels of **HDL** (high-density lipoprotein) cholesterol (the "good" cholesterol – think "H" for happy) **lower the risk** of heart disease. Research has shown that low levels of HDL cholesterol seem to be a stronger risk factor for women than for men.

High blood pressure. High blood pressure is a major risk factor for heart attack and the most important risk factor for stroke. Women have an increased risk of developing high blood pressure if they are obese, have a family history of high blood pressure, are pregnant, take certain types of birth control pills or have reached menopause. African-American women tend to have higher blood pressure levels, increasing their risk for stroke.

Physical inactivity. Various studies have shown that lack of physical activity is a risk factor for heart disease and indirectly increases the risk of stroke. Overall, studies have found that heart disease is almost twice as likely to develop in inactive people than in those who are more active. As we said in Chapter 1, when you're inactive and eat too much, you gain weight. Excess weight can lead to high blood cholesterol levels, high blood pressure. diabetes and increased risk of heart disease and stroke. To control excess weight, see "Simple Pledges for a Physically-Active Lifestyle" on pages 24 & 25.

When needed, a weight loss of just 5 to 10% of your total body weight may reduce your risk of developing diabetes by as much as 50%. Sound like a lot? Consider that if you weigh 200 pounds, 5% is just 10 pounds… that's a great start toward a healthier life!

Simple Pledges...
for a Healthy Heart

I *pledge to:* ✔

❑ Talk to my family about our history of heart disease and stroke.

❑ Eat a balanced diet which is low in fat and high in fiber to improve my heart health.

❑ Find activities I enjoy and get moving!

❑ Stop Smoking!

❑ Understand my risk factors and communicate with my health care providers about regular monitoring of my blood pressure. (Many large pharmacies now offer free blood pressure screening in store.) A healthy blood pressure is below 120 systolic (top number) and less than 80 diastolic (bottom number).

❑ Control my cholesterol through a healthy diet. A healthy cholesterol is below 200 mg./dl.

❑ Know my diabetes risk. If I have diabetes, I pledge to help control it by choosing sugar-free snacks and beverages; eating smaller, more frequent meals; and regularly monitoring my blood sugar levels.

Finally, your first line of defense against heart attack and stroke is to know the warning signs!
See pages 38 & 39.

TAKE A PLEDGE FOR BETTER HEALTH at www.speakingofwomenshealth.com

Obesity and Excess Weight. If you have too much fat – especially if it is located in your waist area – you're at higher risk for health problems, including high blood pressure, high blood cholesterol, high triglycerides, diabetes, heart disease and stroke.

Diabetes. Compared to women without diabetes, women with diabetes have from **two to six times the risk of heart disease and heart attack** and are at much greater risk of having a stroke. People with diabetes often have high blood pressure and high cholesterol and are often overweight, increasing their risk even more.

What Other Factors Contribute To The Risk Of Heart Disease And Stroke In Women?

High triglyceride levels. Triglyceride is the most common type of fat in the body. Research suggests that having high triglycerides may increase the risk of heart disease for women more than for men.

Excessive alcohol intake. According to a recent study published in *Circulation*, the risk of heart disease in people who drink moderate amounts of alcohol (an average of one drink for women per day) is lower than in nondrinkers. However, it's not recommended that nondrinkers start using alcohol or increase the amount they drink. Excessive drinking and binge drinking may contribute to obesity, high triglycerides, cancer and other diseases, raise blood pressure, cause heart failure and lead to stroke. Pregnant women should not drink alcohol in any form.

Heart Of The Matter

It is believed that the heart is where all emotion lives, and that to listen to one's heart is the way to live. Therefore, a healthy heart is essential for healthy living. So, **TAKE A PLEDGE FOR BETTER HEALTH** and start living heart-healthy.

What you should know...

Latest advances in treatment

A simple blood test for heart disease in older women...

According to a new study published in the Archives of Internal Medicine, the white blood cell count could identify post-menopausal women at risk of heart disease. There is increasing evidence suggesting that inflammation plays a key role in heart disease. Markers for inflammation may, therefore, indicate risk for heart disease, even in the absence of other symptoms. A higher white blood count might be an indicator of inflammation.

Still another indicator of inflammation in the body is the CRP, or C-Reactive Protein, also measured through a simple blood test. Ask your doctor if this inexpensive test may be right for you.

Building Blocks...
for Being Heart Smart

Your first line of defense against heart attack and stroke is to know the warning signs! And, they may differ for women.

Heart Attack Warning Signs

Although not portrayed as such in movies, many heart attacks start slowly, with only mild pain or discomfort. Often people affected aren't sure what's wrong and wait too long before getting help. In addition, heart attack symptoms in women may be very different from those in men, and they may be far more subtle.

These warning signs include:
- ✔ Feeling breathless, often without chest pain
- ✔ Flu-like symptoms such as nausea, clamminess, cold sweats
- ✔ Unexplained fatigue, weakness or dizziness
- ✔ Difficulty sleeping
- ✔ Pain in the upper back, shoulders, neck or jaw
- ✔ Feelings of anxiety

If you experience these symptoms, seek medical attention immediately. Don't hesitate to call 9-1-1.

Calling 9-1-1 is almost always the fastest way to get lifesaving treatment. Emergency medical services (EMS) staff can begin treatment when they arrive — up to an hour sooner than if someone gets to the hospital by car. EMS staff are also trained to revive someone whose heart has stopped by performing cardiopulmonary resuscitation (CPR). For more information about CPR, see page 135.

Building Blocks...
for Being Heart Smart

Sudden Cardiac Arrest (SCA)

SCA strikes immediately and without warning. Here are the signs:

- ✓ Sudden loss of responsiveness. No response to gentle shaking.
- ✓ No normal breathing. The victim does not take a normal breath when you check for several seconds.
- ✓ No signs of circulation. No movement or coughing.

If cardiac arrest occurs, call 9-1-1 and begin CPR immediately. If an automated external defibrillator (AED) is available and someone trained to use it is nearby, involve them. And, even if you have never used an AED before...use it now. It's perfectly safe and will not deliver a shock unless one is needed.

Stroke Warning Signs

The American Stroke Association lists these as the warning signs of stroke:

- ✓ Sudden numbness or weakness of the face, arm or leg, especially on one side of the body
- ✓ Sudden confusion, trouble speaking or understanding
- ✓ Sudden trouble seeing in one or both eyes
- ✓ Sudden trouble walking, dizziness, loss of balance or coordination
- ✓ Sudden, severe headache with no known cause

If you or someone with you has one or more of these signs, don't delay!
Immediately call 9-1-1 or the emergency medical services (EMS) number so an ambulance (ideally with advanced life support) can respond. Also, check the time so you'll know when the first symptoms appeared. If given within three hours of the start of symptoms, a clot-busting drug may reduce long-term disability for the most common type of stroke.

Building Blocks...
for Reducing Stress

Stress can be a significant contributor to high blood pressure and heart disease. If you're feeling especially stressed, your body needs...

Vitamin B6
Bananas, figs, prunes, potatoes, chick peas, cauliflower, fortified cereals

Biotin
Soybeans, liver, fish, egg yolks, whole grains

Carbohydrates (unrefined)
All fruits and vegetables, legumes, buckwheat, whole grain foods, brown rice, bran

Fluids
Water, fruit juices, herbal tea

Iron
Dried fruit, dark green leafy vegetables, lean red meats, poultry, seafood, legumes, eggs, fortified cereals

Niacin
Lean meats, fish, canned tuna, legumes, nuts, fortified cereals, whole grain breads

Pantothenic acid
Avocados, broccoli, mushrooms, legumes, meats, whole grain cereals

Potassium
Fresh fruit, dried fruit, prune juice, vegetables, lean meats, seafood, legumes, milk

Building Blocks...
to Protect Against Heart Disease and Diabetes

Vitamin C
Cantaloupe, strawberries, citrus fruits, citrus fruit juices, cranberry juice, tropical fruits, dark green leafy vegetables, cruciferous vegetables (broccoli, cauliflower, cabbage)

Anthocyanins
Berries – blackberries, blueberries, strawberries, raspberries, cranberries, grapes, cherries

Carbohydrates (complex)
All fruits and vegetables, legumes, buckwheat, whole grain foods, brown rice, bran

Chromium
Grapefruit, broccoli, fortified breakfast cereals

Vitamin E
Dark green leafy vegetables; vegetable oils such as cotton seed, peanut, sunflower, and safflower; wheat germ; nuts; seeds; whole grain cereals

Fiber
Fruit (especially with skin), dried fruits, vegetables, cruciferous vegetables, legumes, whole grains and cereals, oats and oat bran products, brown rice

Vitamin B$_6$
Bananas, figs, prunes, potatoes, chick peas, cauliflower, fortified cereals

Lycopene
Tomatoes and tomato products, guavas

Folate
Fruits, dark green leafy vegetables, legumes

Omega-3 fatty acids
Some fish, including anchovies, bluefish, herring, salmon, sardines, trout, canned light tuna; and oils, including canola and flaxseed

Magnesium
Root vegetables, dark green leafy vegetables, seafood, legumes, whole grains, wheat germ, brown rice, nuts, seeds

Mono-unsaturated fats
Avocados, olives, olive oil, canola oil, nuts

Potassium
Fresh fruit, dried fruit, prune juice, vegetables, lean meats, seafood, legumes, milk

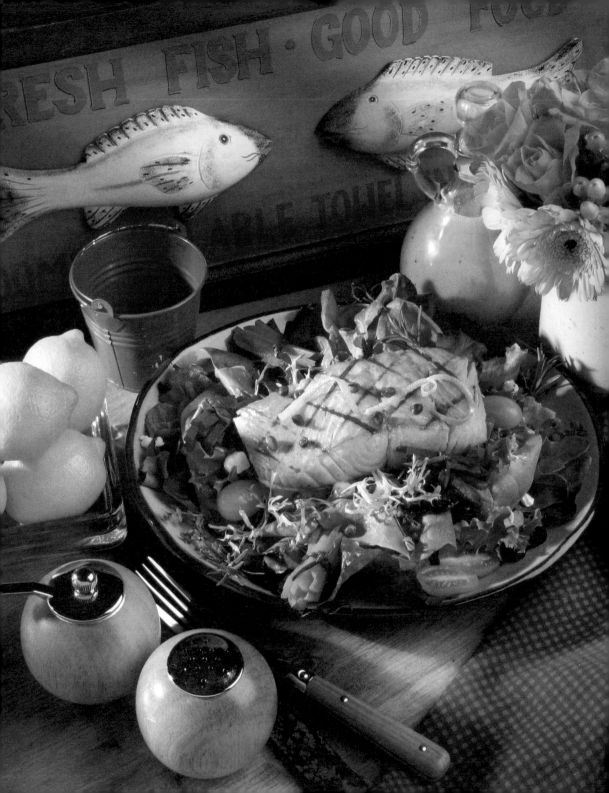

Salmon Salad

Thanks to Mary Wilson of the Supremes
Universal Sisters, National Minority Health Spokesperson

This is a great recipe for leftover grilled salmon (see last year's book, *Recipes for Living Well*, or log on to www.speakingofwomenshealth.com for recipe). Serve over a salad of lettuce, chopped peppers, or vegetables and sprinkle citrus vinaigrette. You've got a quick, easy and delicious meal.

INGREDIENTS

4 oz.	grilled (or baked) salmon
2 oz.	citrus vinaigrette dressing
1 Tbsp.	capers
4	kalamata olives
	colorful, sliced peppers, tomatoes or the vegetables
1 Tbsp.	scallions
1 cup	Romaine or Bibb lettuce

Optional Vegetables
blanched broccoli, carrots or beets

Dressing
½ cup	lemon or lime juice
½ cup	extra virgin olive oil
1 tsp.	minced garlic

Dressing recipe makes approximately four 2-ounce servings

PREPARATION

- Arrange lettuce on plate, top with veggies. Place salmon on top and sprinkle with vinaigrette.

NUTRITIONAL ANALYSIS
Serves: 1
Each serving contains approximately:
292 calories
25 g. protein
7 g. carbohydrates
19 g. fat (1 g. saturated fat)
19 mg. calcium

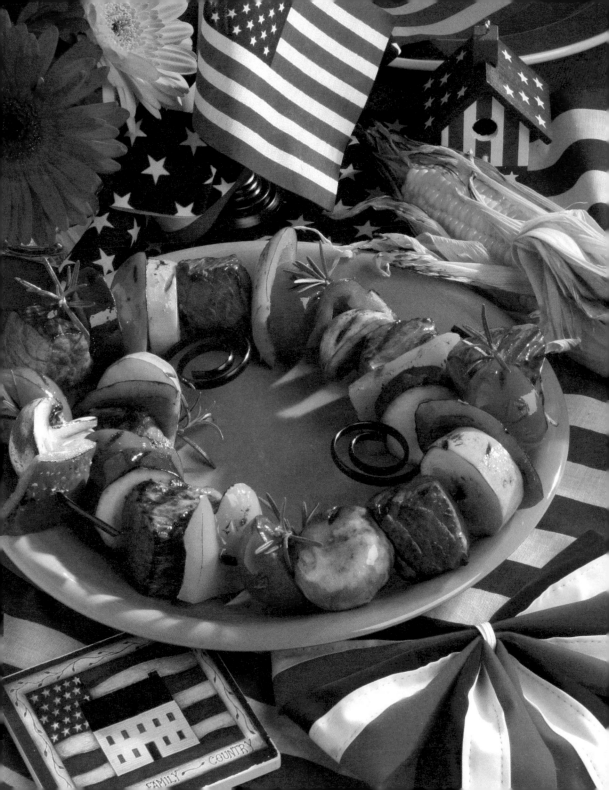

Grilled Kabobs

Thanks to Mark Trowbridge
Merchandise Manager, Neighborhood Market Division, Wal-Mart

What's 4th of July without a backyard grill…and what better to grill than a healthy kabob, full of vegetables fresh from the market or garden! Have fun by substituting mango, pineapple, and tomatoes or try pork, lamb or even chicken…any of your favorites.

INGREDIENTS

1½ lbs. beef tenderloin or grilling steak

assorted vegetables

marinade (store-bought or homemade)

cooking spray

Optional Vegetables
red onions, mushrooms, brightly colored peppers, summer squash, zucchini, grape, cherry or yellow tomatoes

PREPARATION

- Cut marinated meat into 1 ounce chunks.
- Cut vegetables of your choice into large pieces – red onion, mushrooms, grape tomatoes, brightly colored peppers, yellow tomatoes, cherry tomatoes (put this on the end and add it last), summer squash, zucchini.
- Marinate veggies separately from meat.
- Soak wooden skewers in water to keep them from burning.
- Skewer, alternating meat with veggies. Spray with vegetable oil…Grill until meat is cooked thoroughly, rotating position on grill at least once.
- If using cherry or grape tomatoes, add just 1 minute before kabobs are finished cooking.

NUTRITIONAL ANALYSIS
Servings: 3
Each kabob (with three 1 ounce pieces of beef) contains approximately:
268 calories
28 g. protein
15 g. carbohydrates
9 g. fat (3 g. saturated fat)
Fat, cholesterol and calorie content varies with different cuts of beef. Choose lean cuts such as round or beef loin, or trim fat from edges of meat.

Chapter 4
Healthy Bones

"In search of my mother's garden,
I found my own."

— Alice Walker

A simple pledge...

for strong bones begins with something as simple as putting one foot in front of the other. Walking is quite simply one of the best things you can do for building your own strong bones. Surprised…aren't you? Don't be. The best exercise for building strong bones is weight-bearing exercise. And, when you walk, you're bearing your own weight. Now, that's simple! And…it's never too late.

Why are strong bones important? Let's first look at the basics of bone formation. Bone is living tissue that's constantly being renewed in a two-stage process (resorption and formation) that occurs throughout life. In the resorption stage, old bone is broken down and removed by cells called osteoclasts. In the formation stage, cells called osteoblasts build new bone to replace the old. During childhood and early adulthood, more bone is produced than removed, reaching its maximum mass and strength by the mid-30s. After that, bone is lost at a faster pace than it's formed, so the amount of bone in the skeleton begins to slowly decline.

There are several reasons for bone loss which can lead to a disease called osteoporosis. Osteoporosis is a disease that thins and weakens bones to the point where they break easily – especially bones in the hip, backbone (spine) and wrist. Osteoporosis is called the "silent disease" – you may not notice any changes until a bone breaks. But your bones may have been losing strength over many years.

Osteoporosis is incredibly common. A woman's risk of developing it rises with age, especially in the first five to seven years after menopause. During this time, drops in estrogen may result in a 20% loss of bone mass. For women older than 50, the risk of suffering an osteoporosis-related bone fracture is about 50%. Think a broken bone is no big deal? Think again!! Complications from an osteoporosis-related fracture may be so serious as to even lead to death.

Let's Look At The Facts...

Who's at risk for osteoporosis?

✔ Females are more at risk than males.

✔ Those with a small, thin body (under 127 pounds).

✔ Those with a family history of osteoporosis.

✔ Women who are post-menopausal.

✔ Those of Caucasian or Asian race are at greater risk, but African-American and Latino women are also at risk for developing the disease.

✔ Those whose history includes an abnormal absence of menstrual periods; having an eating disorder, such as anorexia nervosa or bulimia that can cause menstrual periods to stop before menopause; and loss of bone tissue from too much exercise.

✔ Men with low testosterone levels.

✔ Those with a diet low in dairy products or other sources of calcium and Vitamin D.

✔ Those with an inactive lifestyle.

✔ Those with a history of long-term use of certain medications (medicines prescribed for many diseases, including arthritis, asthma and lupus); anti-seizure medications; gonadotropin releasing hormone for treatment of endometriosis; aluminum-containing antacids; certain cancer treatments; and excessive thyroid hormone. Talk to your pharmacist to see if your medications put you at increased risk.

✔ Those who smoke and overuse alcohol.

How Do I Know If I Have Weak Bones?

There are tests you can get to find out your bone strength, also called bone density. One test is a dual-energy x-ray absorptiometry (DEXA). A DEXA takes x-rays of your bones. There are also other types of screenings to determine bone mass. Look for free screenings available in your community.

Building Blocks...
for Strong Bones

Get enough calcium each day

Foods are the best source for this important mineral. Supplements vary in the amount of calcium they contain. Those with calcium carbonate have the most amount of useful calcium. Supplements should be taken with meals. Because the body can only absorb so much calcium at once, experts recommend breaking supplements into two dosages, taken morning and evening.

Ages	9-18	19-50	51 and older
Milligrams per day	1000	1200	1300

Get enough Vitamin D each day

Vitamin D is necessary to help you absorb your intake of calcium. You can get Vitamin D through sunlight and foods, like milk. You need 10-15 minutes of sunlight to the hands, arms and face (don't forget your sunscreen!), two to three times a week to get enough Vitamin D. You can also get Vitamin D by eating foods or taking a supplement.

Here's how much Vitamin D you need each day.

Ages	9-50	51-70	71 and older
IU per day	200	400	600

Eat a healthy diet

Other nutrients, like Vitamins A & C, magnesium and zinc, as well as protein, also help build strong bones. **The good news is**, if you follow a healthy diet, low in fat and loaded with fruits and vegetables, you'll achieve success. See Chapter 1 for more specifics.

Think about taking medications to prevent bone loss and reduce fracture rates. See page 51 for more information.

Get Moving

Don't be afraid that exercise may overburden already weakened bones. Being active really helps your bones by:

- ✔ Slowing bone loss
- ✔ Improving muscle strength
- ✔ Helping your balance

Do weight-bearing physical activity, which is any activity in which your body works against gravity and bears its own weight. There are so many things you can do: walk, dance, run, climb stairs, garden, do yoga or tai chi, jog, hike, play tennis, golf or lift weights…it all helps!

Here are some tips on how to start a program of weight-bearing exercise and resistance training that will benefit your bones and muscles and also help your general health.

Weight-Bearing Exercise

For most people who have osteoporosis, brisk walking is ideal. It can be done anywhere, requires no special equipment, and carries minimal risk of injury.

The full benefits of walking come from a regular schedule – at least 30 minutes, three to four days per week. Start at whatever level is comfortable for you. Ten-minute walks are fine at first, but try increasing their length by 1 minute every other time until you reach the optimal exercise level.

Resistance Training

Lifting weights or using strength-training machines strengthens bones all over your body, especially if you exercise all of the major muscle groups in your legs, arms and torso. Strength training is a slow process, so begin slowly and build up gradually at your own pace. For each exercise, select weights or set the machine so the muscle being trained becomes fatigued after 10 to 15 repetitions. As muscles strengthen, gradually add more weight. But don't increase the weight more than 10% per week, since larger increases may raise your risk of injury. Remember to lift with good form, and don't sacrifice good form to lift more weight.

What About Falls?

For many women, the real devastation of osteoporosis occurs when they slip, fall or trip and fracture a bone – usually the hip or an arm or leg bone. The problems are amplified among older women, who may take longer to recover or never fully walk again after a broken hip.

"When a woman has a hip fracture, her death rate is very high," notes Lana Holstein, MD, "because a fracture like that is a trauma that sets up a reaction throughout the body." Older people who are hospitalized with hip fractures may also be at a higher risk to develop life-threatening pneumonia. Osteoporosis is the cause of 1.5 million fractures each year. **TAKE A PLEDGE FOR BETTER HEALTH** today to prevent falls.

✔ Make sure you can see and hear well. Use your glasses or a hearing aid if needed.

✔ Ask your doctor if any of the drugs you are taking can make you dizzy or unsteady.

✔ Use a cane or walker if your walking is unsteady. Wear rubber-soled and low-heeled shoes.

✔ Make sure all the rugs and carpeting in your house are firmly attached to the floor.

✔ Use bathroom aids, including grab bars and stools, to help steady or pull yourself up. In and out of the tub or shower, use bathmats with rubber backing.

✔ Keep your rooms well lit and the floor free of clutter. Use nightlights.

How Is Osteoporosis Treated?

Lifestyle changes and medical treatment are part of a total program to prevent future fractures. These drugs are approved for the treatment or prevention of osteoporosis:

✔ **Risedronate (Actonel®).** This drug is a bisphosphonate and is approved for both prevention and treatment of osteoporosis; for bone loss from the long-term use of osteoporosis-causing medications; and for osteoporosis in men. Actonel is the only therapy proven to significantly reduce fractures of the spine in just one year. Actonel helps to make bones stronger and less likely to fracture by reducing the effect of the cells that weaken bone.

✔ **Alendronate (Fosamax®).** This drug is also a bisphosphonate, approved for prevention and treatment of osteoporosis, and reduction of spine and hip fractures.

✔ **Calcitonin (Miacalcin®).** Calcitonin is a naturally-occurring hormone involved in calcium regulation and bone metabolism. Calcitonin can be injected or taken as a nasal spray. In women who are at least five years beyond menopause, it has been shown to slow bone loss and increase spinal bone density.

✔ **Raloxifene (Evista®).** This drug is a selective estrogen receptor modulator (SERM) that has many estrogen-like properties. It is approved for prevention and treatment of osteoporosis and can prevent bone loss at the spine and hip.

✔ **Parathyroid Hormone or Teriparatide (Fortéo®).** This form of parathyroid hormone is approved for the treatment of osteoporosis in post-menopausal women and men who are at high risk for a fracture. It helps new bone to form and increases bone density.

✔ **Ibandronate Sodium (Boniva®).** This recently-approved osteoporosis drug is taken just once a month, or 12 times a year. It is approved for the treatment of osteoporosis in post-menopausal women.

In addition, estrogen is also FDA-approved to manage osteoporosis and is effective in reducing bone fractures. As with all medications, be sure to discuss with your doctor or health care provider which medication may reduce your risk of osteoporosis-related bone fractures.

Minerals For Life!

New research shows that two minerals…magnesium and phosphorous, may be very important for building healthy bones. Magnesium is believed to be as important to bone health as calcium. Magnesium is found in whole grain cereals and breads; vegetables such as spinach, broccoli and lima beans; milk and yogurt; and lentils, nuts and seeds.

Phosphorous is the body's source of phosphate, which helps create and manage energy, synthesize protein, fat and carbohydrates, contract muscles, and maintain the body's fluid and electrolyte balance. It is also essential for stimulating hormone production and helping the body utilize the B vitamins. It combines with calcium to help form the latticework for strong bones and teeth. More than 80% of the body's phosphorous is located in bone. A proper balance of magnesium, calcium and phosphorous should be maintained at all times.

The good news is that phosphorous is abundant and widely distributed in most foods, therefore there is little chance of a phosphorous deficiency. It is also abundant in many sodas (think phosphate). Your phosphorous intake should equal that of your calcium intake per day.

Simple Pledges...
To Build Strong Bones

I pledge to: ☑

☐ **Eat foods like yogurt, spinach, fortified cereals, salmon and almonds – all are calcium-rich and low in fat.**

☐ **Improve muscle strength through daily weight-bearing exercise such as walking, working with hand weights, gardening or dancing.**

☐ **Increase my balance by stretching my muscles daily to promote greater flexibility, that leads to balance. I may consider yoga or tai chi to help get me started.**

☐ **Stop smoking.**

☐ **Limit my alcohol intake.**

What to eat to build strong bones...

Vitamin A and Beta-Carotene
Sources include deep orange fruits, orange winter squash, carrots, broccoli, dark green leafy vegetables, liver, low-fat milk, eggs

Calcium
Low or non-fat dairy products, broccoli, dark green leafy vegetables, sardines and salmon with bones, calcium-fortified foods

Vitamin D
Fatty fish, such as herring, salmon and sardines, egg yolks, fortified milk and cereals

Vitamin K
Broccoli, Brussels sprouts, dark green leafy vegetables, liver, legumes, eggs

Manganese
Pineapple, sweet potatoes, spinach, chick peas, whole grains, brown rice, nuts, seeds

Phytoestrogens
Flaxseed, edamame (green soybeans boiled in their pods), other soy products

Zinc
Lean meats, liver, seafood, poultry, lentils, whole grains, wheat germ, buckwheat, Brazil nuts

TAKE A PLEDGE FOR BETTER HEALTH at www.speakingofwomenshealth.com

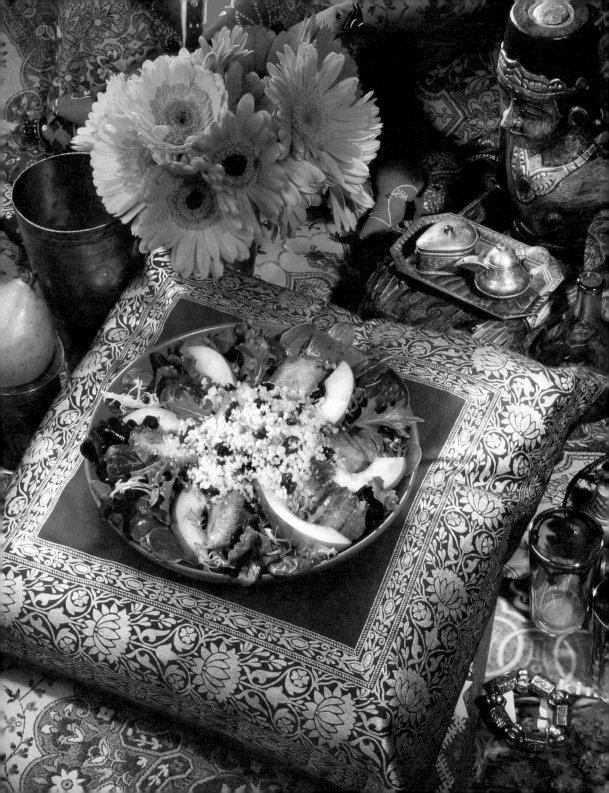

Moroccan Couscous Steak Salad

Thanks to Anthony Hubbard
Manager, Account Specific Marketing, Kellogg's

This is a terrific salad for any occasion, and the flavor of the fruits and spices really is delightful. Use leftover steak, or flank steak (see last year's book, *Recipes for Living Well*, or log on to www.speakingofwomenshealth.com for recipe).

INGREDIENTS

8 oz.	steak, sliced thinly
1 cup	cooked couscous
1 sliced	pear
2 cups	mixed greens
2 oz.	blanched almonds

Dressing

1/4 cup	olive oil
2 Tbsp.	lemon juice (lime works great also)
1/4 cup	raspberry vinegar (any flavored vinegar works, experiment to find your favorite)
1/2 tsp.	sugar

PREPARATION

- Prepare couscous according to package directions, but replace water (liquid) with sugar-free apple juice. Stir in 1 tsp. ground cinnamon and 1/4 cup golden raisins or currants.

- Arrange on a plate:

   Mixed field greens

   Sliced pear

   Blanched almonds or pistachios, to taste

   Thinly sliced steak (served warm or cold)

   Create a bed of couscous in center of plate

NUTRITIONAL ANALYSIS
Serves: 2
Each serving, with 4 oz. steak and 1/2 cup cooked couscous, contains approximately:
410 calories
32 g. protein
44 g. carbohydrates
13 g. fat
22 mg. calcium

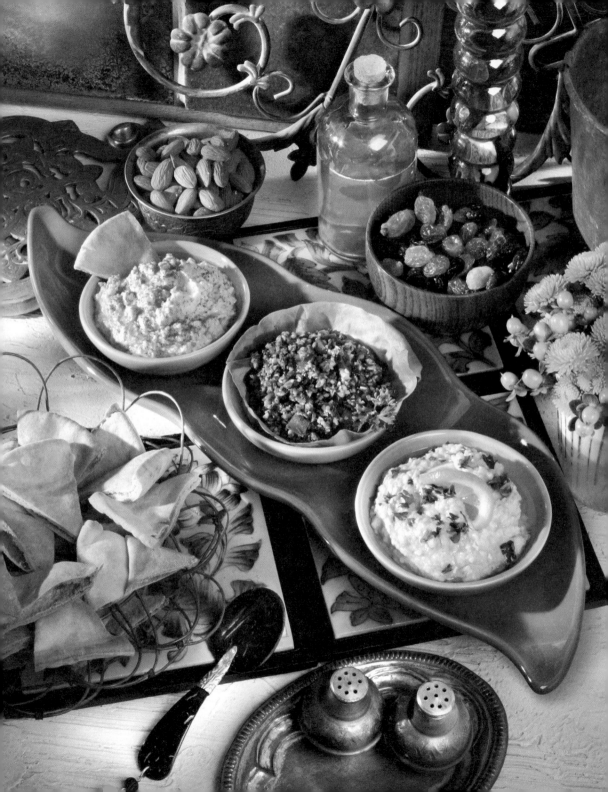

Hummus
Traditional and with variations

Thanks to Radhika Saveri
Marketing Manager, Stouffer's Lean Cuisine

Hummus has become a very popular dip – it is low in fat, vegetarian and full of protein. Try it with variations, or the traditional way on a toasted pita wedge, baked tortilla or your favorite whole-grain cracker. It's also a great-tasting and healthy alternative to mayonnaise on a burger!

INGREDIENTS

2 cups	chick peas, soaked and cooked or canned, drained and rinsed
3 Tbsp.	lemon juice
1/4 cup	water
3 Tbsp.	tahini (sesame paste)
dash	olive oil
	parsley and lemon slices

Variations – Consider adding

1/2 -1 tsp.	cumin
1/2 tsp.	paprika
1/2 tsp.	cayenne pepper
1/2 cup	roasted peppers (process together with chick peas)
1/2 cup	eggplant (cook until tender, peel and cut into chunks and process together with chick peas)
3 cloves	roasted garlic

PREPARATION

- Place the cooked chick peas (it's ok if they're still warm) in the food processor along with the garlic, lemon juice and water. Process for about a minute, until smooth. If too thick, add more water.
- Stir in the tahini and spices.
- Spread the hummus into a shallow bowl, drizzle with olive oil, and garnish with lemon slices and minced parsley.
- Serve chilled, with warm pita bread and/or fresh vegetables.

NUTRITIONAL ANALYSIS
Serves: 8
Each serving contains approximately:
109 calories
5 g. protein
12 g. carbohydrates
3 g. fat
30 mg. calcium
Hummus is also high in magnesium, potassium, phosphorous (see page 52) and folate!

Chapter 5
A Balanced Life

"My formula for living is quite simple. I get up in the morning and I go to bed at night. In between, I occupy myself as best I can."

—Cary Grant

A simple pledge...

for a balanced life begins
with giving yourself the
gift of a few moments each day
to nourish your soul.

The ultimate in better living, for many of us, is achieving BALANCE! Finding that right mix of mind, body and spirit; home, work and family; friends, career and relationships; whatever your challenge...Balance can sometimes seem like an unattainable goal. **The good news is**...while it may seem impossible... it's not!

What's The Secret?

Balance begins with perspective. Some women believe that within each day, the hours must be equally balanced for life to "work". Not so, say both Dr. Deb Kern and life coach Jennifer Lewis-Hall, both national keynote presenters for Speaking of Women's Health. "We cannot think about balance in the context of a single day, or even a month. The key is to look at life in its entirety," says Lewis-Hall, author of *Life's a Journey, Not a Sprint.*

In our 20s, schedules are often dominated by work, sometimes school or education, and relationships. In our 30s, we may have demands of young children, marriage and a growing career. Then come our 40s, when many of us are challenged to find balance between guiding our children, who are becoming young adults with their own lives, aging parents who require more care, our own changing bodies and our evolving relationships...add to that a career and the realization that it's time to plan for retirement...and, balance may seem like something achievable only for "other people". In our 50s, our children often leave home to begin their own families, but that doesn't mean suddenly we've got the world on a string. Now, we may feel pulled to do even more, to work more, focus on our relationships more, spend time with grandchildren, and, often we may find ourselves caring for an elderly relative. And, then, of course there's that slight distraction happening, called menopause!

"It's important to look at a span of time to find out if life is balanced," adds Dr. Kern. "And, much of balance comes from within. As women, we have to put ourselves at the top of our own to-do lists! If we don't have energy and vitality, we certainly cannot take care of others."

Balancing Time For You
Our Speaking of Women's Health readers, and those women who attend our conferences, tell us that it's true. Stealing 20 or 30 minutes a day to do something for yourself actually gives you more energy and helps you feel like you have more time in your day! Doctors and health care providers agree that when you take the time to exercise each day, you actually accomplish more.

Balancing Stress
Balancing stress is also a reality. Some stress is inevitable, and, if handled well, may be motivating. But, for those times that you feel overwhelmed by pressures and demands for your time, whatever else you do...don't forget to take care of yourself. As women, it's not uncommon to stay up late just to get those last few things off your list. That's fine once in a while, but when it becomes the norm, it can become a problem. Working through lunch is another strategy for many women. Again, this isn't a problem if you keep some healthy snacks at your desk or even drink a nutritional supplement in place of your meal. But, not eating throughout the day may cause your blood sugar to drop, which creates foggy thinking, fatigue, mental instability and lack of alertness. **Nutritionists also suggest bringing a healthy lunch from home, last night's left-overs heat up nicely in the office microwave...and so do healthy frozen meals.**

Simple Pledges...
for Putting Yourself First!

I pledge to: ☑

☐ Practice deep breathing exercises for at least 5 minutes.

☐ Join, or create a book club.

☐ Take a few minutes at the beginning and end of each day to pamper my skin...cleanse, tone, moisturize and protect.

☐ Take a class from the local community center, Y or church. Consider yoga, knitting, welding, scrapbooking or a spiritual study.

☐ Ask my family to prepare at least one dinner each week. I will use the time to take a bubble bath or go for a walk. Then, I will arrive at the dinner table as if I'm a guest.

☐ Invite some girlfriends for a slumber party. Why not? After all, I loved it when I was younger! See page 141 for some fun slumber party inspiration.

☐ Take 5 minutes before I leave work to think about the evening ahead...and relax before picking up the kids or greeting my spouse.

Simple Pledges...
to encourage a Body-Mind-Spirit Balance!

I pledge to: ☑

☐ Eat well	☐ Sleep well	☐ Move my body
☐ Enjoy my work	☐ Touch	☐ Practice Deep Breathing
☐ Nurture my relationships	☐ Find a spiritual connection	☐ Laugh

TAKE A PLEDGE FOR BETTER HEALTH at www.speakingofwomenshealth.com

Balancing The "Blues"

It's important to realize that, for many women, feeling stressed or out of sync may be just "the blues". However there are times when depression may be more serious and even life-threatening. **The good news is** today, our health care professionals have some great tools to help us deal with depression, anxiety and other types of mood disorders.

When To Seek Help

According to Walter Smitson, PhD, Professor, Department of Psychiatry, University of Cincinnati College of Medicine, President & CEO, Central Clinic, Inc., it's vital to know when to seek help. Here are some guidelines, but use your own judgement:

✔ When feelings of depression persist for more than two weeks.

✔ When serious depression interferes with your daily activities. Signs of depression include loss of interest in daily activities, diminished appetite, difficulty concentrating, changes in sleep patterns and feelings of guilt or worthlessness. You may want to consult with your pastor or spiritual advisor, family counselor or professional.

You may also discuss it with those you rely on for support – family, friends, children, co-workers. **The good news is**...up to 80% of those who seek treatment will notice rapid improvement, usually within a few weeks. Often lifestyle modifications may help get your life back on track. Consider these:

✔ Limit your caffeine to just a few cups a day. Caffeine may boost your mood temporarily, but you may feel a letdown once it wears off.

✔ Get enough calcium. Research suggests that calcium may help with mood swings often associated with Pre-menstrual Syndrome (PMS). And, it's also great for your bones and plays a role in weight loss. (See page 53 for good sources of dietary calcium.)

When you invite balance into your life, you inevitably help those around you find balance. Yoga instructors refer to this as putting out "good karma". An everyday way to think about this is if others around you are happy and in balance, you will reap those rewards in return. One person at a time, one family at a time, one community, one country, one continent, one world...think of it as a ripple effect. Setting your own priorities and finding your personal life balance could actually affect world peace. On those busy nights at home, wouldn't you settle for family peace?

Building Blocks...
for Balance

Pledge to succeed! Have a set schedule and routine to help keep on track. Implement a family calendar, color-coded for each family member.

Put things into perspective. Decide what's important for you and your family and build your priorities around those things. Family game night may mean a lot more to your kids than a sparkling clean house...figure out what works for your situation.

Keep healthy finances. Put your family on a budget and stick to it. Set aside what you can for emergencies and for future needs, including retirement. Pack lunch rather than buying. When shopping, look for better values. Join frequent flyer and hotel chain clubs and bank your points earned for future travel.

Get your B's!! Research indicates that many depressed adults are lacking sufficient nutrients, including Vitamins B_6 and B_{12}. Both B_6 and B_{12} vitamins help protect long-term mental health and regulate mood. Consider a supplement if your diet alone isn't sufficient.

Exercise daily! Activity boosts levels of chemicals in the brain that elevate mood. Even a short walk can help. See Chapter 2 for all of the advantages of fun physical activity.

Get some fresh air and sunshine! Exposure to sunlight triggers the release of melatonin in the brain, which regulates your sleep and wake cycles and can have a powerful effect on energy and mood. As always, use a SPF (sun protection factor) of 15, or a moisturizer containing sunscreen.

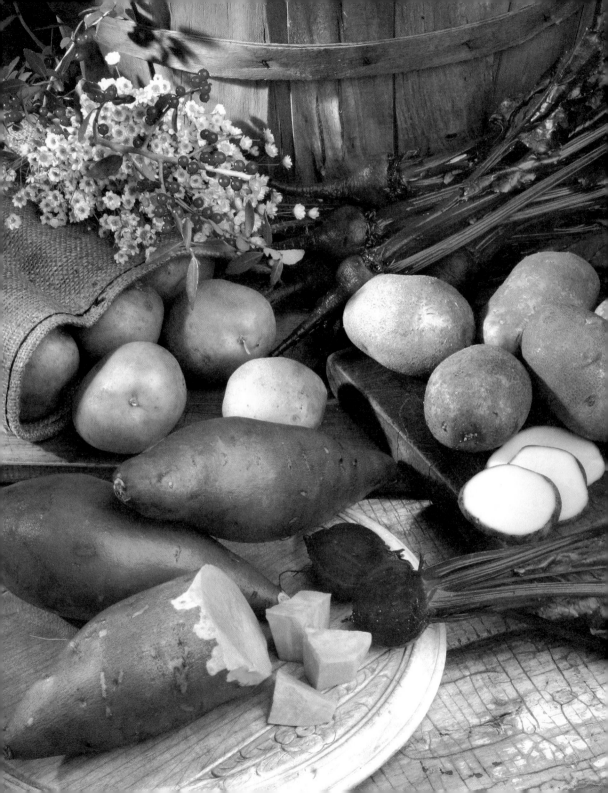

Colorful Mashed Potatoes

Thanks to Lynn Picard
Executive Vice President / General Manager, Lifetime Television Network

We love to experiment with mashed potatoes. Try adding roasted garlic, fat-free sour cream, or low-fat cheese for added flavor. Experiment with different types of potatoes such as Yukon Golds or Peruvian Purples for a different flavor. Or, have fun with colors with the variations below.

INGREDIENTS

1 lb.	potatoes, peeled and quartered
2 quarts	water
¼ cup	low-fat (1%) milk
	salt and pepper to taste

Variations

Leave the skin on the potatoes for added texture, flavor and fiber.

"Pink" potatoes

Substitute ½ pound beets for ½ pound of the potatoes. Boil beets and potatoes together, then mash together with other ingredients.

"Orange" potatoes

Substitute sweet potatoes for regular potatoes. Peel after boiling. Prepare as directed.

PREPARATION

- In a medium saucepan, bring the water to a boil. Add the potatoes, then bring the water to a simmer for 20 to 25 minutes, or until the potatoes are tender. Remove the pan from heat and drain the water.
- Add the milk, salt and pepper.
- Use a mixer to combine the ingredients until they are smooth.
- Serve immediately.

NUTRITIONAL ANALYSIS, with potatoes
Serves: 4
Each serving contains approximately:
104 calories
4 g. protein
20 g. carbohydrates
1 g. fat

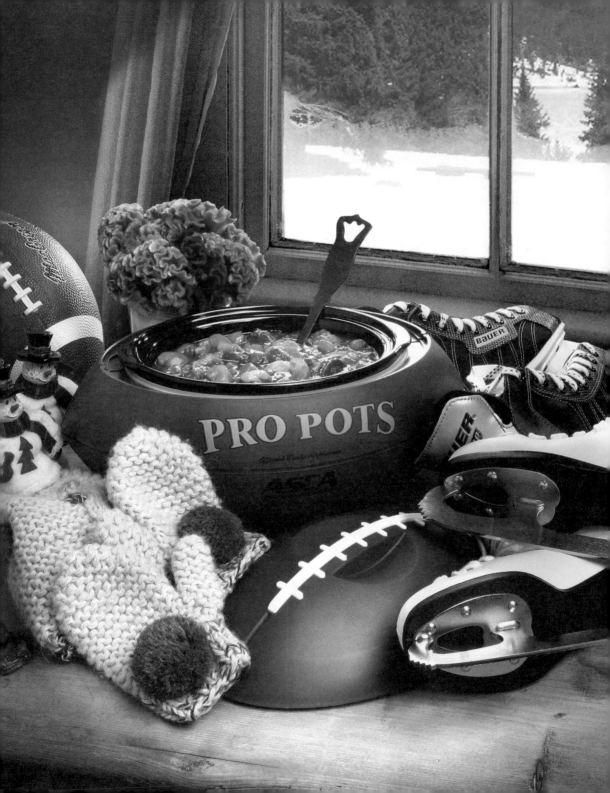

Beef Stew

Thanks to Keisha Scott
Corporate Marketing Manager, Wal-Mart

Beef Stew is a hearty meal for chilly nights, and this recipe works great in a slow cooker, which is a terrific time saver. Your family will love coming home to the aroma of dinner ready-to-eat! Who'll know you weren't in the kitchen all day?!

INGREDIENTS

2 lbs.	stew beef
4 large	carrots, sliced
1 cup	celery, sliced
2	onions, diced
1 can	water chestnuts, sliced
2 Tbsp.	tapioca
1 cup	red cooking wine
1 cup	mushrooms, sliced
1 tsp.	sugar
1 large can	whole tomatoes, coarsely chopped

PREPARATION

• Put everything in a small roasting pan, cover and bake at 325 degrees for 4 hours.

Optional
Consider serving over rice or noodles

NUTRITIONAL ANALYSIS
Servings: 8
Each serving contains approximately:
201 calories
24 g. protein
7 g. carbohydrates
8 g. fat (2 g. saturated fat)
54 mg. calcium

Chapter 6
Hormones
From 15 to Fabulous!

"For attractive lips, speak words of kindness.
For lovely eyes, seek out the good in people.
For a slim figure, share your food with the
hungry.
For beautiful hair, let a child run his or her
fingers through it once a day.
For poise, walk with the knowledge you'll never
walk alone."

— Audrey Hepburn

A simple pledge...

for celebrating the stages of your life begins with
appreciating yourself and an understanding of how to
communicate where you are physically and how
you're feeling emotionally to your friends,
family and health care providers.

One of the most interesting things about being a woman is that life is never boring…we go through lots of changes. We love to change our clothing, our looks, our tastes, and…our minds. What's not always fun is when our hormones play havoc and "change" our moods.

The fact is that from the onset of puberty until well beyond menopause, women have hormonal fluctuations which some tell us…"rival the rise and fall of the oceans themselves"! The question is, how do these hormones affect us, physically and mentally? A great deal of research has been conducted on the physical effects of hormones. Finally, science is beginning to understand the key role hormonal fluctuations may play in how women metabolize medicines, what symptoms may be present for heart disease and stroke (cardiac and vascular disease), and how we age. Only recently has science begun to investigate the role of hormonal fluctuations on a woman's libido.

If you feel that the quality of your life's energy is being compromised, you're not alone! We now know that improper balances of estrogen, progesterone and testosterone may negatively impact a woman – emotionally, physically, and, even sexually.

When we talk about libido, most of us think immediately of sexual desire…actually, this is just one part of our libido, or "life's energy". Energy for life fuels our vitality and nourishes our souls, filling us with zest and drive to be productive, energetic and power-full women. And, yes, libido also provides us the desire for intimacy and sexual fulfillment. If you're lacking desire or energy for life…sexually, physically and even emotionally…your hormones may be the culprit.

There is a lot of information available about ways to measure and treat hormonal imbalances, and what options may be available to help put energy back into your life and some passion into your relationships.

Our Common Ground

Whether we're 15, 50… (or, even more "Fabulous"!), as women, there's one thing we all have in common… hormones! There's no question that our hormonal fluctuations impact our thoughts, feelings, behaviors and moods. BUT…the question is… *how are you going to manage it?*

At one time or another, we've all blamed something on "raging hormones" – a bad case of acne, a bout with depression, lack of energy or sexual desire or even weight gain. But what exactly are hormones? They're the body's chemicals that regulate everything from strength and growth to moods and sexual development.

The female sex hormone is estrogen. It's produced by the ovaries, and without it, a girl can't reach sexual maturity (she won't ovulate or develop breasts).

Testosterone is the pilot of male sexuality. It's produced in the testicles, and without it, a boy can't reach his sexual maturity (his voice won't deepen, and he won't grow facial or body hair).

Did you know that women, too, have a natural supply of testosterone, but in much smaller quantities? As women, our challenge with the effects of low testosterone doesn't typically begin until after menopause, when our bodies' natural hormone supplies diminish. Post-surgical menopause may also trigger these effects, along with severe weight loss due to anorexia or excessive exercise which causes menstruation to stop.

Hormonal effects go beyond mood swings. Hormonal imbalances have been linked to increased risk of breast and uterine cancers, heart disease, obesity, loss of bone mass, fatigue and sleep disorders. Poor diet and lifestyle choices, stress and medications, can also magnify the negative effects of hormonal imbalance. See page 73 for Simple Pledges to help take charge of your changing body and hormones. Let's take a closer look at what's happening in our bodies…

PMS

For many women, pre-menstrual syndrome (PMS) begins in their 30s. For others, it may begin far earlier. Symptoms, which crop up as early as two weeks before your period and generally stop when it starts, are wide-ranging and may include some of the following: bloating, weight gain, breast tenderness, headache, backache, acne, irritability, depression, anxiety and

Take charge of your changing body and hormones. You, and only you, have the power to decide if you're going to "Keep Your Life Power Full" or let your hormones rule your world.

fatigue. Studies show that PMS is not only the result of hormonal changes, but also is caused by changes in the brain's chemicals, including serotonin.

Talk to your doctor if PMS symptoms become more than you are comfortable with. The selective serotonin reuptake inhibitor (SSRI) antidepressants can manipulate these brain chemicals and relieve symptoms. Used at half-strength and only in the last two weeks of your menstrual cycle, SSRIs work largely by making more serotonin available to the brain.

Peri-Menopause

Peri-menopause is the phase before menopause actually takes place, when ovarian hormone production is declining and fluctuating, causing a host of symptoms.

Here's what you may expect:

✔ Your once-predictable cycle is starting to lose its clockwork regularity, thanks to hormonal changes.

✔ Your period may come more frequently. Bleeding may be heavier and last longer, for six or even seven days.

✔ Your hormone system is beginning to misfire at times. Production of both estrogen and progesterone begins to be less predictable, affecting your body's messages to your brain.

Don't be surprised if you experience some of these symptoms during peri-menopause: hot flashes, insomnia, fatigue, irritability or mood swings, unusual weight gain, irregular periods, anxiety, feelings of depression, fuzzy thinking, bloating or gas, headaches, joint pain or stiffness, vaginal dryness, diminished sexual desire and leaking of urine. *Take heart…no one has all of these symptoms.*

Simple Pledges...
for Living with Hormonal Fluctuations

I *pledge to:* ☑

☐ Exercise, three to five days per week, to improve my mood and decrease PMS symptoms.

☐ Look for low-sodium nutrition choices to help minimize bloating and swelling.

☐ Eat a healthy diet rich in complex carbohydrates and low in simple sugars.

☐ Decrease my caffeine and alcohol intake to reduce irritability, mood swings and breast discomfort.

☐ Take part in relaxation techniques, such as meditation or yoga, to decrease physical discomfort and stress.

☐ Drink a minimum of 8 glasses of water each day to prevent dehydration, which aggravates PMS symptoms.

TAKE A PLEDGE FOR BETTER HEALTH at www.speakingofwomenshealth.com

Menopause

Literally, menopause means "pause of menses", or the menstrual cycle. For most women, the average age of the last menstrual period is 51, although menopause itself can begin as early as the 30s and last beyond the age of 51. A woman is considered to be "post-menopausal" when she's gone a full year without a menstrual period. Menopausal symptoms are the same as those listed previously for peri-menopausal symptoms.

The loss of estrogen means that a woman's health and appearance can undergo profound changes. As estrogen wanes, a woman's risk of heart disease increases, as does her risk of osteoporosis, and urinary tract changes that can lead to incontinence or cause more frequent urinary tract infections. In addition, some women may notice that their skin is no longer as supple as it once was. **The good news is**…most women, by paying attention to the important issues of exercise, diet, mental activity and self-care, are better prepared to meet these challenges head on.

For some women, menopause is a big deal. For others, it's a barely noticeable shift from the child-bearing years into years of "post-menopausal zest" and discovery.

Since the beginning of time, menopause itself hasn't changed, but the lives of women certainly have. At the turn of the 20th Century, the lifespan of the average woman was 48, meaning many women never even made it to menopause. By contrast, today's woman can expect to live well into her late 70s, a statistic that puts millions of women into what is known as the "post-menopausal years". The average woman, in fact, will spend one-third of her life beyond menopause, no longer concerned with a monthly menstrual period or pregnancy, but now facing some of the health challenges that come with aging and maturity. Even when you're post-menopausal, you still need to have regular pelvic/gynecological exams. This is the time when many women become more at-risk for certain gynecologic cancers, and regular exams are your best defense!

What women should understand is that menopause is totally natural. It's a stage of life…a transition from one phase to another. It is *not* an illness that needs to be treated or fixed. Today's women have far more information and knowledge about their bodies and what to expect of the menopausal years, and **the good news is** that some very self-directed decisions can make profound differences in how women experience this new phase of life and health. Educate yourself about all of the options, so you can make the best choices about how to manage the symptoms of menopause, how to protect from diseases brought on by loss of estrogen, and how to be the person you'd like to be.

Living With Stress Incontinence

Stress incontinence has nothing to do with "emotional stress". The term refers to urine leakage during any physical activity that results in increased pressure on the abdomen. This pressure need not be much: bending over, laughing and coughing can cause urine leakage in stress incontinence sufferers. Many people suffer silently, too embarrassed to seek help. **The good news is** that treatment for urine leakage is readily available.

Maintaining appropriate weight, exercising, and drinking enough water are vital for healthy living. There are also effective ways to improve bladder control. Treatment of incontinence usually starts with exercises to tone pelvic muscles and retrain the bladder. These are called Kegel exercises. Drug therapy may include prescription estrogen or non-hormonal medications. Minimally-invasive surgical procedures now exist for the treatment of urinary incontinence. A frank discussion with your doctor, urologist or uro-gynecologist will be your best path to recovery.

Because urinary problems are embarrassing to women, some never seek help for a very treatable condition. But, help is available for this very common, but often under-discussed, problem.

Building Blocks...
for Controlling Incontinence

✔ It's easy to assume that drinking less fluids will lead to fewer wetting accidents. Unfortunately, it's just not true. Lack of fluids can lead to constipation, which also puts pressure on the bladder. Cutting down on fluids isn't the answer.

✔ By all means, drink the eight glasses of water you need to stay hydrated. Avoid excessive use of caffeinated beverages. Caffeine is a natural diuretic – even one cup of coffee will increase urine production.

✔ Some fruit and vegetable juices, such as tomato and grapefruit, may aggravate existing bladder problems.

✔ Consider meeting with a qualified dietician, who can advise you on beverages and food groups to avoid.

Embracing Change

Let's face it…we all have our "days"! "Whether it's monthly PMS, menopausal symptoms or post-partum changes…it's up to you to decide how to live with these ever-present mood swings and physical symptoms. You can certainly take responsibility for your actions, and not allow yourself to be emotionally hijacked by your hormones. How often have you heard someone make an excuse for rude behavior or disinterest and blame it on PMS…or just a sour mood? Is that how you want to be thought of? Learn to embrace responsibility and be the person you'd like to be every day…not just on good days. Put a smile on your face and communicate positive, friendly and supportive messages even when your body may not be at it's best. Keep your sense of humor intact!" These words of wisdom come from Speaking of Women's Health national speaker, Robin Smith, PhD.

Hormones aside, if you desire a stronger relationship with your spouse, children, family, friends, co-workers, neighbors…a good place to start is with your SELF. The healthiest relationships we know exist between the people who are most "at-home" with themselves. The key to building strong relationships begins with your own relationship with your SELF. That means appreciating WHO you are, HOW you look, WHY you react to certain things the way you do and WHEN you need something. Once you learn to respect and honor yourself, then you can reach out to others.

PMS got you feeling moody and irritable? Ever wonder why you crave chocolate just before your period? It turns out that chocolate is a mood enhancer. Chocolate contains phenethylamine (PEA), which stimulates the nervous system, triggering the release of endorphins that dull pain and give a sense of well being.

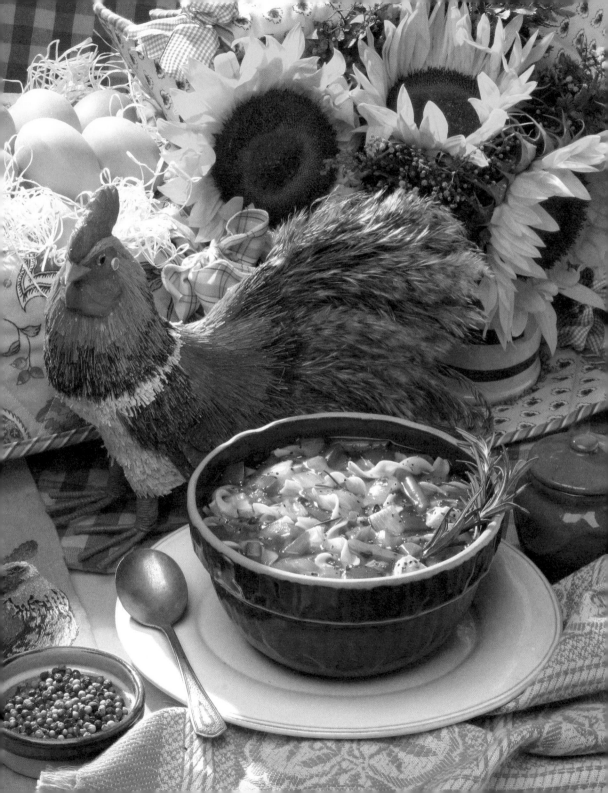

Chicken Soup

Thanks to Adrienne Sapp
Corporate Marketing Manager, Wal-Mart

Hormonal fluctuations may leave you craving comfort food, and nothing's better than tasty chicken soup just like Grandma's. Enjoy!

INGREDIENTS

4 lbs.	fresh chicken
2 quarts	water
3	stalks of celery, coarsely chopped
3	carrots, coarsely chopped
1 large	onion, coarsely chopped
	small bunch of herbs, tied together (may include thyme, parsley, bay leaf, and savory teas.)
	peppercorns to taste
2 cups	green beans
1 cup	red bell peppers, chopped

Optional
cooked noodles or
cooked brown rice

PREPARATION

- Place chicken in stock pot.
- Add all the remaining ingredients except the onion, green beans and red bell pepper, and bring to a simmer.
- Simmer uncovered for about 3 hours. Skim any fat or grease that may develop on top.
- Remove the chicken, clean the meat from the bones. Dice the meat and reserve. Discard the bones.
- Discard the bunch of herbs.
- Refrigerate the stock and remove the fat from the top after it cools.
- In a stock pot, combine cooled chicken stock, reserved chicken and reserved vegetables.
- Add 1 large onion, finely chopped, green beans and red bell pepper.
- Salt and pepper to taste.
- Reheat.

NUTRITIONAL ANALYSIS
Servings: 6-8
Each 1½-cup serving contains approximately:
236 calories
11 g. protein
11 g. carbohydrates
17 g. fat (4 g. saturated fat)

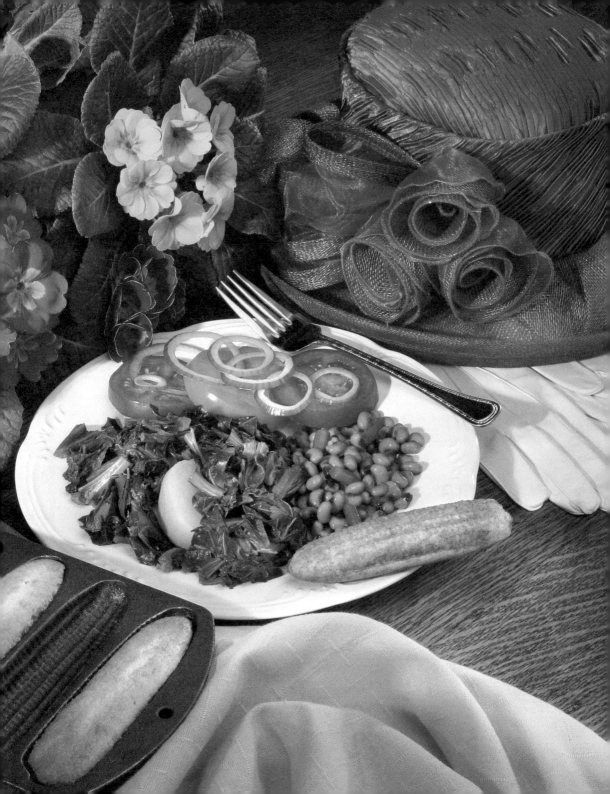

Vi's Sunday Greens

Thanks to Linda Flournoy
Writer, Editorial Department, Creative Studio, American Greetings

This recipe comes straight from Linda's Mom, who loves to cook greens on Sunday. We think they're a perfect addition to any table! Greens are loaded with calcium, iron and vitamins! Enjoy them anytime!

INGREDIENTS

1	onion, chopped
1 lb.	fresh turnip greens (with or without turnip roots attached)
1 lb.	fresh kale greens
1 lb.	fresh mustard greens
1½ lbs.	fresh spinach greens
3 small	or 2 large smoked turkey tails
1	whole garlic clove
1 Tbsp.	olive oil
	salt and pepper to taste

PREPARATION

- Thoroughly wash greens in cool water.

- Peel and cut turnip roots into quarters.

- Rinse and place smoked turkey, garlic, turnip roots, and olive oil into a 5-quart pot, fill with water, cover, and bring to a rapid boil for 15 minutes.

- Add turnip, kale and mustard greens to boiling water.

- Reduce to medium heat, cover and cook 1 hour.

- Add spinach, and cook for 15 minutes.

Prior to eating, some may prefer to discard the turkey tails.

Serve as a meal or side dish. Garnish with sliced tomatoes and sweet onions.

NUTRITIONAL ANALYSIS
Servings per recipe: 4
Each serving contains approximately:
59 calories
3 g. protein
5 g. carbohydrates
4 g. fat (0 saturated fat!)
4 g. fiber
115 mg. calcium

Chapter 7
Beauty and
Healthy Skin

"Though we travel the world over to find
the beautiful, we must carry it with us or we
find it not."

— Ralph Waldo Emerson

A simple pledge...

for beauty begins with a daily
commitment to cleanse, tone,
moisturize and protect your skin.
How easy is that!

For all that has been said about beauty over the years, and all that has been written, created and manufactured to "create" or represent beauty...the most basic form of beauty is what our grandmothers told us from the beginning...*Beauty begins from within.* Beauty is the reflection of one's inner spirit. And, a spirit full of passion for life, joy and confidence creates a striking reflection in the mirror.

Add to that reflection a bright smile, and you're sure to find beauty. A smile is the most important accessory you can put on. It is contagious...when someone smiles at you, you can't help but to smile in return.

As women, we don't separate how we look from how we feel. We've all had "bad hair days" or those mornings when nothing in our closet fits right and we just want to crawl back into bed and not face the world. Well, chances are...that's not an option! When we look good, we feel good...and, when we feel good, our self esteem soars. When we're feeling confident, we want to share that with the world, and we're more likely to take better care of ourselves.

Like the rest of your body, your skin undergoes some changes as you age. You may begin to notice fine lines and wrinkles around your mouth and eyes. You may notice that the texture of your skin is not as smooth as it once was. Maybe, it has uneven tone and dullness, enlarged pores, dryness, blotches and age spots. Some women even experience acne...again! **The good news is**...there's plenty you can do about it!

Simple Pledges...
for a Beautiful You

Looking and feeling your best means taking care of yourself inside and out. In addition to a healthy outlook on life, here are some simple pledges to help put "nature's roses" on your cheeks.

I pledge to: ☑

❑ Drink plenty of water.

❑ Get enough sleep.

❑ Stop smoking, because smoking damages skin, especially the delicate area around the eyes and mouth.

❑ Maintain a physically-active lifestyle.

❑ Eat a balanced diet, low in fat and full of fruits and vegetables.

❑ Establish a simple daily skincare routine...cleanse, tone, moisturize and protect.

❑ Protect myself from the sun's harmful rays, the number one cause of skin damage and wrinkling. I will use a sunscreen with a minimum SPF (sun protection factor) of 15 on all exposed areas of skin each and every day and consider a daily moisturizer or foundation with sunscreen added.

❑ If I can't live without that "healthy glow" of a tan...I will use a sunless tanning product and avoid tanning beds and "laying out".

TAKE A PLEDGE FOR BETTER HEALTH at www.speakingofwomenshealth.com

Sun Safety And Beauty

Try these simple tips to use sunscreen correctly and to protect yourself and your family. Doing so may help you significantly reduce your risk of skin cancer, and wrinkles that make you look older than you are.

✔ Always use a sunscreen with a minimum SPF of 15. Apply 15 to 30 minutes before exposure. Reapply every 2 to 3 hours, whether you're using a waterproof sunscreen or not.

✔ Choose a sunscreen product that is convenient, easy to use, and that you find pleasant to apply. Why is this important? Studies show that if you like the smell, for example, or the way it feels on your skin, you are more likely to reapply sunscreen often, providing greater protection for your skin. So, whether it's a cream, oil, spray, gel or any combination thereof…choose a product you like and use it! Many products are specially-formulated for sports activities, for children, for sensitive skin or for faces…so, you've got plenty to choose from.

✔ Limit your time in the sun. Avoid the sun when it's hottest, typically between 10 a.m. and 4 p.m. Don't be fooled by cloudy days…up to 70% of the sun's rays penetrate cloud cover. And, reflective surfaces can increase your risk of burning. Watch out for concrete, sand and snow.

✔ Wear protective clothing and sunglasses. Be certain children wear a hat with a wide brim, to protect their head and eyes. Consider adding a t-shirt for added protection.

✔ Ask your pharmacist if medications you're taking may increase your sensitivity to sunlight and increase your risk of sunburn.

✔ Avoid using harsh products or chemicals on your skin. Moisturize all over after bathing to seal in your skin's own moisture. Choose well-tested and researched national brands, with a toll-free number on the packaging.

Did you know that up to 80% of skin's damage from the sun occurs before the age of 18? Start a lifelong habit with your children, or grandchildren, with sunscreen. Teach them to protect themselves from the sun's harmful rays. On average, children get three times as much sun exposure as do adults.

4
Building Blocks to Beauty

First, it's essential to develop a skincare routine that's simple and "do-able". Here's an easy 4-step process for healthy skin:

CLEANSE
Use a mild cleanser specially-formulated for your skin type – normal, dry, oily or sensitive. Do this morning and evening.

TONE
Daily toning removes excess oil and impurities and helps maintain skin's natural PH balance.

MOISTURIZE
New products are designed to address your skin's unique needs. Look for daytime products that work under your make up and nighttime formulas for more moisture.

PROTECT
Again...Use sunscreen every day to protect from the sun's rays.

Beyond Beauty

The most serious danger to sun exposure is skin cancer. Carcinomas are the most prevalent skin cancers. They range from flat, scaly red areas (basal cell carcinoma) to raised, ulcerated tumors (squamous cell carcinoma) to the least common, but most deadly skin cancer, malignant melanoma. Because it begins in moles or in the skin's tanning cells, it's important that you know the **ABCDs** of danger:

✔ **A**symmetrical shape,

✔ **B**orders that are irregular or jagged,

✔ **C**olors that are mixed or uneven,

✔ **D**iameter that is more than one-quarter inch.

No one is immune to the sun's cumulative effects. Although people with fair skin, light hair, and blue eyes burn most easily and are more susceptible to acute effects of sun exposure and damage, those with dark skin also face risks. Risks can be minimized with a few healthy habits.

Enhancing Your Natural Beauty

✔ Take advantage of today's cosmetics to enhance your natural beauty. Experiment with foundations or tinted moisturizer to even skin tone, and concealers to hide imperfections. Choose a color palette that matches your skin tone, hair color and what you're wearing. But, don't get so caught up in color rules that you don't allow yourself to have a little fun experimenting with different shades and types of cosmetics. For daytime wear, choose light shades that enhance your natural look. For evening, add some drama with metallics or brighter tones.

- ✔ Look for double-duty products. For example, choose a lipstick that moisturizes and protects lips.

- ✔ Invest in good quality brushes and applicators. Replace when worn or soiled. Do not share any applicator used on or around the eye. Potentially-harmful bacteria or virus may be spread this way. Always wash hands before applying make up.

- ✔ Make sure to keep your make up clean and stored properly when not in use, and kept in a moderate temperature range away from extreme cold and heat. Following these simple rules will help to keep your make up bacteria-free and help it to last for its maximum time.

Beautiful Foods For Beautiful Skin

New research suggests that a healthier diet may have a complexion connection. New studies suggest that a diet loaded with fruits and vegetables may also help reduce wrinkling. It may be the high content of antioxidant vitamins like A, C and E and phytochemicals found in those foods. These foods include carrots, winter squash and pumpkin, citrus fruits, canteloupe, berries (strawberries, blueberries, raspberries taste great on your morning cereal or mixed with low-fat yogurt for a healthy snack), cruciferous vegetables (broccoli, cauliflower, cabbage), dark green leafy vegetables, nuts, seeds, whole grain cereals and low-fat dairy foods.

Remember how much fun you had as a child creating "art"? Think of cosmetics as the color for your canvas (skin) which will allow you to create your masterpiece. Have fun choosing your "day" look, your "evening" look and your "professional" look.

Women Of Color

Women of color have special skincare problems and needs, and luckily the personal care industry has responded with new products in recent decades. Manufacturers now create entire lines of cosmetics – foundations, powders, blushes, eye shadows, etc. – for women of color whose skin tones are dark, olive or blended.

Each skin type, in fact, has its own characteristics:
Afro-Caribbean Skin tends to be thicker, has good elasticity and healthy levels of oil, and tends to age slowly.

Asian Skin is slightly thicker than Caucasian Skin and because it has lots of melanin, ages slowly.

Latin Skin texture and color vary considerably and tends to be oily.

And regardless of the coloring or amount of pigment in the skin, women of color are reminded to add sunscreen to their daily routines, because skin cancer affects all shades of skin. White skin is more prone to skin cancer, but dark skin is also at risk for developing cancers.

Beauty...For Life!

Want that "fresh off the beach" look...the safe way? Consider a sunless tanning product. Today's formulas provide plenty of options for you to achieve an even, streak-free, natural-looking "tan", without the harmful effects of the sun's rays. Whether you prefer to apply a spray, lotion, cream or even towelette formula, sunless tanning can leave your skin with a natural-looking glow of color, smooth and soft from added moisturizers.

According to the American Academy of Dermatology, the most effective products available are sunless, or self-tanning lotions that contain **dihydroxyacetone** (DHA) as the active ingredient. DHA is a colorless sugar that interacts with the dead cells located in the stratum corneum of the epidermis. As the sugar interacts with the dead skin cells, a color change occurs. This change usually lasts about five to seven days from the initial application. What a fun, safe way to get your "sugar fix".

Every day, millions of dead skin cells are sloughed off or worn away from the surface of your skin. In fact, every 35 to 45 days, you have an entirely new epidermis. This is why tans from sunless, or self-tanning lotions, will gradually fade – as the dead cells are worn away, so is your tan. For this reason, most products suggest that you reapply the sunless, or self-tanner about every three days to maintain your "tan".

Creating A Halo Effect

Just as with your skin, it's important to choose hair products that are formulated for your hair type – normal, oily, dry or color-treated. There are products that are also designed to compensate for other issues. These may provide a boost of color for natural or color-treated hair, treat dandruff or flaky scalp, provide intense conditioning for weekly use or very light conditioning for everyday use, help rid hair of product build-up, provide sun protection or protect from chlorine when swimming, or add volume, control frizz or add spunk to curly hair. With so many choices, it's easy to find a solution!

"What's important for hair care is to maintain its health, and that begins with an adequate daily intake of protein, B vitamins, zinc and iron. If your hair is nourished and cared for with proper diet, good cleansing and moisturizing, you'll have strong, healthy hair. And, healthy hair is beautiful hair," according to Lydia Evans, MD, dermatologist and skincare expert.

The good news is, what's good for the rest of the body is also what creates the building blocks for healthy, shiny, strong and beautiful hair.

The good news is, what is good for the rest of your body…all of the things we've discussed throughout this book…is also what creates building blocks for healthy, shiny, strong and beautiful hair. This includes a healthy, nutrient-rich diet (specifically loaded with B vitamins and proteins…see sources in Chapter 1), plenty of water, exercise, relaxation, smoking cessation, sun protection and a daily hair care regimen.

Have Fun With Hair Color!

Whether gray hair is making you feel older than you'd like, or if your natural color is screaming for a boost…or, if you just want to have some fun…at-home hair color is a great place to start! Level 3 coloring products are permanent, meaning they don't wash out. Level 2 products are semi-permanent, meaning they wash out in about 28 shampoos. Level 2 products will provide a boost of color, but will not dramatically lighten hair color. Want to try a different shade but confused by all of the choices? The secret to de-coding hair color is simple…use this as a guide.

For Lighter Skin Tones

Choose hair shades with "cool tones" that contain more red than yellow. Light skin tones look best with hair colors that are blond or light brown with natural tones like mahogany.

For Medium Skin Tones

Check out shades close to your natural base with added golden or coppery tones. Go for shades with definitive golden or copper in all the blond, honey brown and intense red tones.

For Darker Skin Tones

Go for warmer shades with dark golden or mahogany tones. Choose shades with golden, mahogany, deep coppery gold, deep coppery mahogany or even rich coppery brown tones.

Be sure to read the instructions and information for each product. Follow the instructions and call the manufacturer's toll free hot-line if you have questions. Also, be sure to conduct a skin allergy test first, before using.

Thinning Hair Is Aging Hair

Many women think thinning hair is not normal, or that it's a man's problem. Some believe that, if their hair is thinning, they must be sick. Temporary conditions such as pregnancy, menopause, medication, diet, or stress can cause hair thinning. But 70% of women who experience hair loss can attribute it to heredity.

The Thinning Process

As you age, heredity, combined with the effects of hormones and age, cause certain hair follicles to get smaller and smaller. This prevents the hair from fulfilling its regular growth process.

Hair Thinning And Ethnic Women

Hair thinning is non-discriminating, meaning that it can happen to all of us regardless of our ethnic backgrounds. In addition to hereditary hair thinning, many African-American women experience other forms of hair loss, which may be due to the use of hair reshaping products (relaxers, straighteners, hot combs) or hair braiding methods.

Taking Action

What can you do to safely regain control of your appearance and make your hair thicker, fuller and easier to style? Depending on the stage of the hair thinning process, there are three options:

1. Minoxidil (2% topical solution) to reverse the thinning process and help stimulate hair growth
2. A wig or hairpiece
3. Hair transplant surgery

What Causes Gray Hair?

Despite what you may have been told, gray hair doesn't happen because of stress or worry. "Graying" is caused because the pigmentation process stops. What can you do about it? Color it!

Building Blocks...
for Styling Thin Hair

✔ Gently massage scalp for 30 seconds each time you shampoo to promote circulation.

✔ Apply a light conditioner to hair ends, rather than at the roots.

✔ Try products specially-formulated to plump up fine hair by retaining moisture.

✔ Choose lightweight styling products that won't weigh hair down.

✔ Apply a little extra styling product to roots for added volume.

✔ When blow drying, towel dry hair first. Don't use highest heat setting.

✔ If you wear a ponytail, avoid using rubber bands.

✔ Try an above-the-shoulder, layered cut to add fullness.

✔ Color or highlight your hair a shade lighter to make hair look full.

Tough As Nails

Have you ever wondered why you cannot wear colored nail polish into surgery? It's because your nails tell a great deal about your overall state of health, including how much oxygen is in your blood – a vital sign closely monitored during a medical procedure.

Nails are composed of minerals and **keratin,** a type of protein. Nails provide protection for your fingertips and are meant to be strong yet flexible, smooth and glossy. Nail health relies on sufficient supplies of protein, B Vitamins, Vitamin A, calcium, zinc, iodine and iron. When your body isn't receiving enough of these vital nutrients, or doesn't absorb or assimilate them properly, the deficiency may surface on your nails. Abnormal or unhealthy nails may also be the result of injury, a glandular deficiency such as hypo-thyroidism, or a deficiency of certain nutrients. Did you know that frequent hangnails may indicate an inadequate supply of Vitamin C, folic acid and protein?

Friends For Life

Give yourself a hand…set aside a little pampering time. Make a pact with a friend to give yourselves a manicure once every two weeks.

We've been cautioned for years to think of our nails as "Jewels, not Tools"! Proper nail care is needed not just so you look good, but is also part of a healthy hygiene routine. Even if you prefer your nails short and natural, a manicure will keep them clean and free from bacteria. Want a fun, pampering treat? Why not get together with your friends for a manicure party. While you're at it, try a pedicure, too…after all, our feet carry the weight of the world!

Hereditary hair thinning is a common part of life for 1 out of every 4 women. Hair loss affects self-esteem.

Women may feel…

- *embarrassed or devastated*

- *less feminine or less attractive*

- *less likely to succeed in business*

- *socially unacceptable or helpless*

- *like they are losing their youth*

- *less desirable*

The good news is…it doesn't have to be that way! See page 91 for solutions.

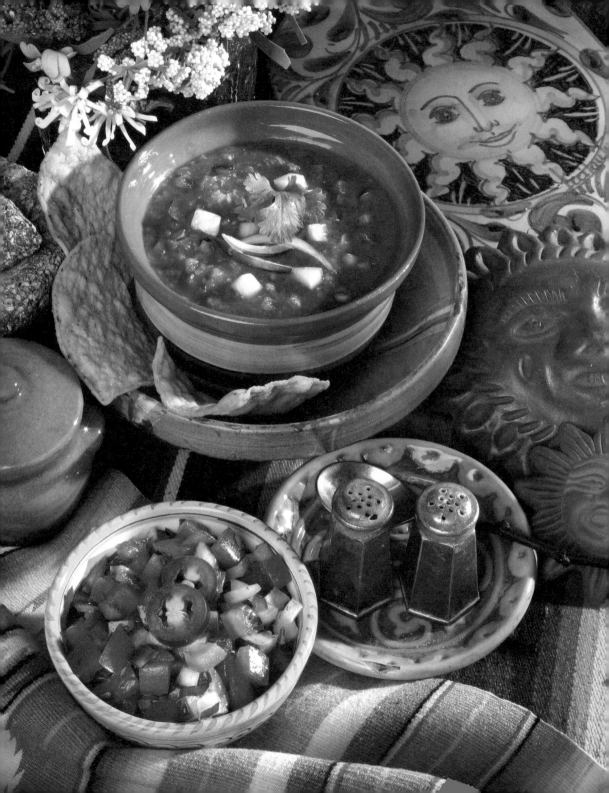

Traditional Gazpacho

Thanks to Allison Wrobel
Associate Brand Manager, Cadbury Schweppes Americas Beverages

Gazpacho is served chilled, which makes it perfect for a summer meal starter. It's low in calories and almost fat-free. Enjoy!

INGREDIENTS

4	ripe, red tomatoes, coarsely chopped (if canned, choose low-sodium, peeled)
1 each	green and red bell pepper, cored, seeded and coarsely chopped (set aside 2 Tbsp. for garnish)
1	cucumber, peeled, seeded and finely diced (set aside 2 Tbsp. for garnish)
1/2	medium red onion, finely diced (set aside 2 Tbsp. for garnish)
2	cloves garlic, chopped
1 slice	french bread, diced
1/4 cup	chopped, fresh herbs, such as basil, oregano and/or flatleaf parsley (set aside 2 Tbsp. for garnish)
1	green jalapeno pepper for garnish
1 cup	ice water, or as needed
2 Tbsp.	extra virgin olive oil
2 Tbsp.	balsamic vinegar, or to taste
	salt to taste
	freshly ground black pepper

PREPARATION

- Process all ingredients together until soup is the desired texture.
- Taste for seasoning.
- Chill for at least one hour before serving.
- Garnish with chopped bell peppers, cucumber, whole basil leaves, red onion, parsley and green jalapeno.
- Pepper, if desired.

NUTRITIONAL ANALYSIS
Serves: 6
Each 1 cup serving contains approximately:
46 calories
7 g. protein
4 g. carbohydrates
2 g. fat (0 saturated fat)

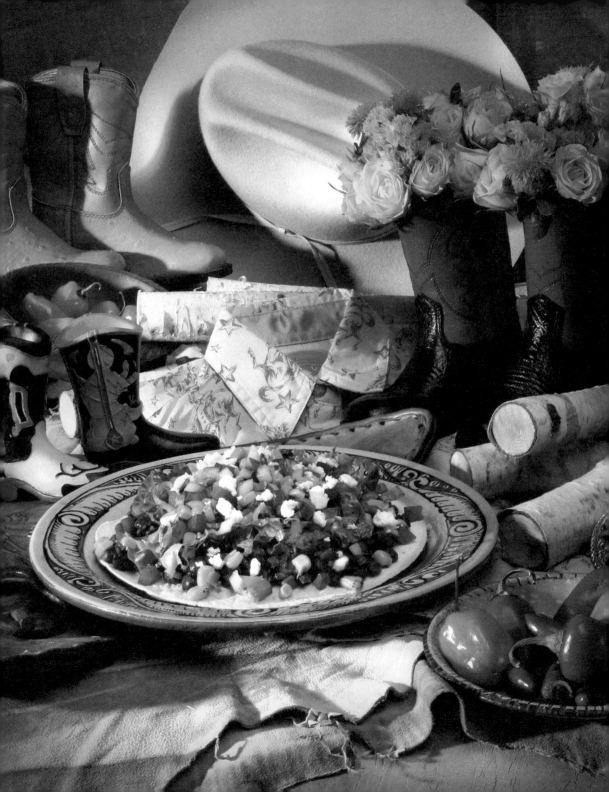

Chalupa

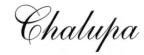

**Thanks to Monica Hysell
Vice President, Medical Nutritional Sales
Ross Products Division / Abbott Laboratories (Ensure)**

Chalupas make a great light meal or cut into wedges for a hearty appetizer. The family will love them, and the **good news is**…they're loaded with veggies and nutrition!

INGREDIENTS

6	whole wheat tortillas
1-14 oz. can	black beans
6 oz.	shredded low-fat cheddar cheese
	grated lettuce
1-14 oz. can	drained low-sodium tomato chunks
1½ cup	salsa

Variations

shredded or ground lean beef, pork or chicken, taco seasonings

canned corn

avocado, cut in chunks

low-fat sour cream

PREPARATION

- Heat tortillas in oven or microwave, according to package directions.
- Lay tortillas flat on a cookie sheet.
- Add ingredients, beginning with a base layer of beans, then tomato, lettuce, any variations and finally top with salsa and cheese.

NUTRITIONAL ANALYSIS, without variations
Serves: 6
Each chalupa (1 tortilla) contains approximately:
276 calories
14 g. protein
29 g. carbohydrates
9 g. fat (6 g. saturated fat)
313 mg. calcium

Chapter 8
Trust Your Gut!

"If you can walk, you can dance.
If you can talk, you can sing."

—Zimbabwe Proverb

A simple pledge...

for trusting your gut begins with listening to what your body's telling you. How difficult is it to make a pledge to "listen"? Listening is the first part of being a good communicator. Listen first...your body will tell you what it needs. Your digestion goes through quite a long pathway, and, it starts with what you put into your mouth.

The terms used to describe common stomach ailments may be a little confusing – gastrointestinal distress, heartburn, digestive problems, upset tummy – they cover a lot of ground! The key is to understand what your "gut" is trying to tell you and to listen and respond appropriately to its signals.

Many experts believe that the "gut" may be your "second brain". Why? There are more neurotransmitters in the 20 feet of your "gut" than there are in your brain! So, those butterflies in your stomach or that feeling in your gut may actually be a legitimate mind/body connection. So, when that voice inside you is speaking... LISTEN! Frequent abdominal distress is a signal that something needs to be addressed.

The good news is...armed with education, lifestyle changes, diagnostic screenings and new and powerful medications....we've got many tools to work with!

Taking Your Pledge For Comfortable Digestion

In its simplest terms, our digestive system is a series of tubes and valves that leads to the stomach and then eventually through the organs that eliminate what our bodies cannot use. As we eat the food, chewing and swallowing it, the food travels to the stomach, where acids and chemicals break it down so that it can pass into the intestines, where key nutrients are absorbed into the bloodstream. Food that's chewed in the mouth enters into the esophagus, a muscular tube about nine inches long. At the top of the esophagus is a small valve that relaxes to let food enter the esophagus and also to keep it from going where it's not supposed to go, or "down the wrong pipe". At the bottom of the esophagus is a stronger valve that relaxes to let food into the stomach. This valve is also known as the lower esophageal sphincter. This sphincter normally prevents the backflow of stomach contents into the esophagus. Many patients with frequent heartburn, also known as gastro esophageal reflux disease (GERD) have been found to have inappropriate, brief relaxations of this sphincter. These relaxations allow the irritating acids and digestive juices of the stomach to come into contact with the esophageal lining.

The effective operation of our digestive system depends on many factors, everything from the amount of acid in our stomach, to our stress levels, to what we eat and when...even what we're wearing when we eat. This may be a simplified version of a very technical biological process, but intestinal distress runs the gamut from mild discomfort caused by occasional overeating to chronic heartburn to even life-altering ulcers or irritable bowel syndrome. The bottom line is...it's not a subject to be taken lightly or to be ignored. Far too many of us don't pay attention to what our "gut" is telling us. Fewer than 25% of those who suffer weekly from intestinal symptoms actually seek medical treatment. The real problem here is, not only do chronic sufferers miss out on a myriad of new treatments to bring relief, but, some may actually overlook a serious illness and chalk its symptoms up to "upset tummy".

GERD

Gastro esophageal reflux disease (GERD) is the abnormal reflux of stomach contents, including acid, into the esophagus (the tubular structure that connects the mouth to the stomach). GERD can manifest itself in many different ways. The majority of people with GERD experience a burning sensation in their upper abdomen after eating, commonly known as "heartburn".

Approximately 7% of the U.S. population experiences GERD-type symptoms daily and roughly 40% of people have GERD on a monthly basis. Numerous tests can confirm the diagnosis of GERD, however the presence of typical symptoms is usually sufficient to make the diagnosis and begin treatment. It should be mentioned that patients with a history of heart disease or with heart disease risk factors (older age, diabetes, smoking, high blood pressure and/or history of heart disease in family members) might need a formal evaluation to establish that the discomfort is not the result of heart problems.

The Most-Common Medicines

Over-the-counter antacids such as Tums®, Maalox®, Rolaids®, Pepto Bismol® and Mylanta®, neutralize the acid in the stomach and are good for relieving symptoms quickly. The liquid forms may work fast, but tablets may often be more convenient. The effect of these antacids may not last long, so repeating doses may be required for relief.

Over-the-counter and prescription H₂ blockers, such as Pepcid AC® and Zantac® work by blocking histamine receptors (that's what H_2 stands for). These receptors stimulate the production of the stomach acids, and by blocking them, the stomach makes less acid, reducing the likelihood of heartburn.

Proton Pump Inhibitors (PPI), such as the newer over-the-counter (Prilosec OTC®) and prescription drugs (Prilosec®, Prevacid® and Nexium®), are powerful substances that block or suppress acid production in the cells that "pump" acid into the stomach. Some studies also have found that PPIs can decrease heartburn-related symptoms, including shortness of breath, hoarseness, chronic cough and laryngitis. *Remember, these are medications in pill form, and not an actual pump.* Once the drugs are at work, they can relieve or prevent symptoms for up to 24 hours.

Other prescription drugs, such as so-called prokinetic medicines that help heal the painful swelling in the esophagus, are typically prescribed for long-term use. Other drugs can speed up digestion, keeping food in the stomach for shorter periods of time, so that reflux has less of a chance to occur, while still others can protect the mucous lining of the esophagus to keep it healthy and functioning.

As with all drug treatments, talk with your pharmacist about risks, benefits and possible side effects.

Simple Pledges...
To Prevent Painful Heartburn

I pledge to: ☑

❑ Not eat just before bedtime.

❑ Chew gum or suck on hard candy after eating to stimulate the flow of saliva, washing juices back into the stomach and helping to neutralize the acid.

❑ Avoid overeating by eating several small meals throughout the day to avoid overfilling the stomach.

❑ Maintain a healthy weight and regular physical activity.

❑ Take a walk after my evening meal to relax and allow my digestive process to begin before settling in for the evening's activities.

❑ Stop Smoking. Tobacco irritates the esophagus and weakens the esophageal sphincter, which causes heartburn and GERD.

❑ Avoid excessive alcohol and caffeine.

❑ Avoid wearing tight-fitting clothing, particularly at the waist. Be certain my pantyhose or jeans aren't too tight, particularly when eating.

TAKE A PLEDGE FOR BETTER HEALTH at www.speakingofwomenshealth.com

In severe cases of GERD or hiatal hernia, doctors might have to perform surgery to repair the valves that control the flow of contents and acid between the stomach and esophagus.

Up, Out & Away!

Okay, who hasn't experienced gas? As "mature" as we get, the thought often elicits giggles or brings to mind embarrassment. For millions of adults, it's no laughing matter. The fact is, on average, our bodies produce one to three pints of gas daily, and we pass it, on average, 14 times a day. Gas is produced in three ways:

1. by the air we swallow when we eat, drink and even talk;
2. by stubborn foods such as carbohydrates which may be difficult for our bodies to digest; and
3. through bacteria that move from our colon to our small intestine.

What can you do to reduce gas and bloating?

✔ Identify the foods that cause you difficulty. Some offenders may include beans, cabbage, Brussels sprouts, broccoli and asparagus. These contain a sugar called raffinose, a major trigger of gas. It's important to realize that these foods may cause a problem occasionally. If one of these foods is a constant source of pain for you, talk to your pharmacist about precautions you can take when you eat this food.

✔ Many starchy foods (including potatoes, wheat and corn) produce gas during digestion. Rice, however, does not, which is why pediatricians tell Moms to feed it to their children who have upset stomachs or diarrhea.

A Word About Chocolate...

For some people, chocolate may be a trigger for GERD. If this is the case, and you need your chocolate, Robin Miller, MD, suggests eating a <u>small piece</u> of chocolate, instead of a <u>small box</u>.

Keep it moving! Exercise tones the intestines and tissues that keep digested food moving through the body. Try taking a walk after meals or on a regular basis. Even something as simple as a walk can get muscles moving in a more "normal" pattern.

Constipation is a common problem that can cause discomfort, bloating and pain. Constipation generally refers to stools that are infrequent, dry or hard, or difficult to pass. Unlike conventional thinking, there is no "right" number of daily or weekly bowel movements. It's important to understand what your "normal" schedule is, and what is regular for you. This regularity may vary slightly depending on what you eat, how active you are and other factors, but in general, you should maintain a fairly regular schedule.

Many Factors May Affect Your Regularity
Women may be affected by hormonal changes brought on by pregnancy, the menstrual cycle and menopause. **Some medicines may trigger constipation,** including antidepressants, pain medications, antihistamines and calcium or iron supplements. Talk to your pharmacist if you take these medications regularly, to determine if you need to take action to help avoid the discomfort of constipation.

To maintain regularity, doctors recommend eating a diet rich in fiber (25 to 35 grams daily), drinking plenty of water and maintaining physical activity. It's not difficult to get the recommended fiber amounts in your daily diet. A breakfast cereal fortified with fiber, 6 daily servings of fruits and vegetables, and a healthy snack of dried fruit or a handful of almonds will hit the mark.

Fiber is an essential part of a healthy diet. Fiber adds bulk to the diet and helps stool move easily out of the body. This is especially helpful for people with constipation. In addition, fiber adds substance to the stool, which can help clear up diarrhea. Friendly bacteria in the intestines love fiber and use it as a food source. A diet high in fiber will also help the good bacteria to grow and protect us from the harmful bacteria.

Some excellent food sources of fiber include… multi-grains, cereals, breads, cinnamon, raspberries, mustard greens, collard greens, broccoli, celery, red chili peppers, fennel bulb, grapefruit, cauliflower, cabbage, green beans, eggplant, strawberries, split peas and lentils.

It is important to increase your fiber intake gradually, over the course of several weeks. Any sudden change in diet may bring on temporary discomfort. Also, increase your water intake to help aid in the processing of the fiber while your body adjusts.

If you need to add a fiber supplement, several over-the-counter remedies are available. Talk to your pharmacist.

Irritable Bowel Syndrome (IBS) – Dysfunction Junction

If you've ever had Irritable Bowel Syndrome, it can be as nasty as it sounds. It usually means that women experience abdominal pain or discomfort and accompanying changes in bowel patterns.

For some, loose stools and frequent bowel movements may become the norm. For others, diarrhea develops and never seems to go away, while some women develop constipation.

Once gallbladder disease or cancers have been ruled out, and a diagnosis of IBS has been determined, a plan for treatment can be developed. **The good news is**…that lifestyle and dietary changes can typically bring about tremendous relief.

According to Christine Lowry, M.Sc., RD, "Fiber is an important component of a healthy lifestyle. It can assist in weight management and help reduce the risk of certain cancers and heart disease, which is the No. 1 killer of women. Despite its many well-known benefits, however, many women still don't get enough fiber on a daily basis."

Simple changes that can keep IBS at bay:

✔ Keep a diary of what factors bring on symptoms.

✔ Try relaxation techniques or hypnosis to calm the entire body and restore normal bowel movements and functions.

✔ Professionals at the International Foundation for Functional Gastrointestinal Disorders point out that if using medicines, they should be used in conjunction with other lifestyle changes, not in place of them.

If you've had a sudden change in your bowel habits, or if you notice blood in your stool, this could be a serious warning. See your doctor. Although it may be nothing serious, these and other changes could be a sign of cancer or other severe illness. Any change accompanied by weight loss, severe pain or bloating requires a call to the doctor.

Colon Cancer

Facts: Colon cancer, also called colorectal cancer, is the third most common cancer in women (and men). Like several other cancers, it's often a "silent" disease because it may exist without symptoms. However, it is a very preventable cancer because early detection and removal of polyps in the colon and rectum may prevent the development of cancer.

Symptoms:
- Rectal bleeding, blood in the stool
- Change in bowel habits
- Cramping pain in the lower abdomen

Early Detection: The tests used to screen for colorectal cancer have strange-sounding names, such as sigmoidoscopy, colonoscopy, barium enema and fecal occult blood tests. Basically, they're all tests that either examine the insides of the colon and rectum to look for polyps (tissue growths) or test for signs of blood in the stool. Once a woman turns 50 (and sometimes earlier), she needs a screening exam for colon cancer. The most thorough screening is a colonoscopy (the gold standard), which many gastroenterologists and colorectal surgeons feel should be repeated every 5 years, if normal. It may be repeated sooner if an abnormality is found. A baseline screening is recommended at age 50. This screening is a great investment in yourself. *Those with a family history of colon cancer need to be tested earlier.* Some doctors believe that African-Americans may be at higher risk for colon cancer.

Building Blocks
for *Living with* GERD

Too much of a good thing... Limit Trigger Foods!
Some foods naturally contain more acid than others or, once eaten, trigger acid production in the stomach. Do you know which ones are troublesome for you? Keeping a food diary will help you pay attention to foods that are most likely to set off your heartburn symptoms. Try to avoid them in the future.

Trigger Foods!
Common foods linked to heartburn may include the following:

- ✔ Coffee
- ✔ Carbonated beverages
- ✔ Peppermint or spearmint
- ✔ Whole milk
- ✔ Fatty or spicy foods
- ✔ Citrus fruits
- ✔ Tomatoes
- ✔ Onions

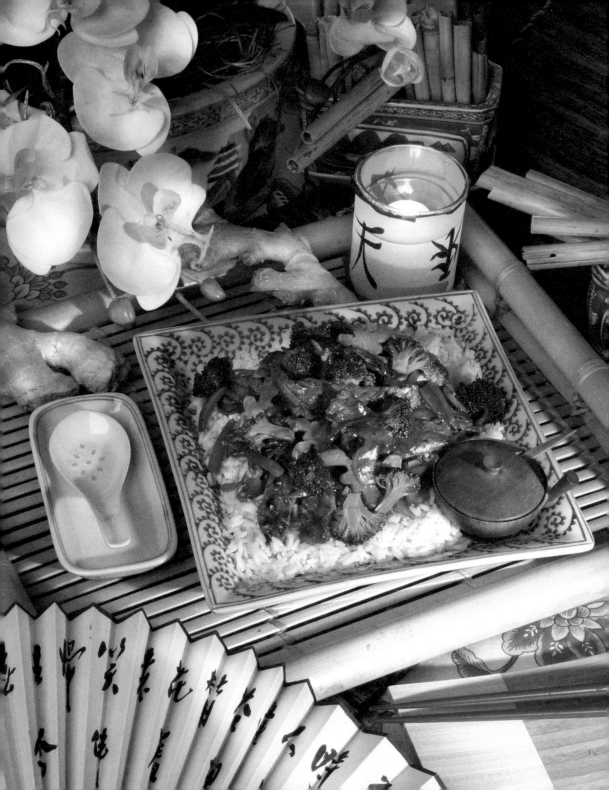

Beef & Broccoli with Ginger

Thanks to Karen Fondu
President, Maybelline New York/Garnier

This Asian-inspired quick and easy meal is sure to please the whole family. Ginger is a tummy tamer, and it tastes great! Serve over brown rice.

INGREDIENTS

1 lb.	sirloin beef, pounded and sliced thin
1 Tbsp.	fresh grated ginger (1 tsp. if powdered)
2 Tbsp.	olive oil
1 large	onion, sliced thin
2 cloves	garlic, sliced thin
1 cup	beef bouillon (low sodium)
1 Tbsp.	sugar
2 Tbsp.	soy sauce (low sodium)
1 Tbsp.	cornstarch
⅓ cup	water
2 cups	thinly sliced/chopped broccoli, including stems
2 cups	cooked brown rice

PREPARATION

- Mix ginger with beef.
- Heat oil in skillet until hot, fry meat quickly. When pink is gone, add onion and garlic. Lower heat.
- Add bouillon, sugar and soy.
- Just before serving, add cornstarch dissolved in ⅓ cup water. Stir.
- In separate pan coated with cooking spray or lightly oiled, stir fry broccoli for 6 minutes or until desired tenderness.
- Serve dish over rice.

NUTRITIONAL ANALYSIS
Servings per recipe: 4
Each serving, with ½ cup cooked brown rice, contains approximately:
413 calories
30 g. protein
34 g. carbohydrates
19 g. fat (5 g. saturated fat)
53 mg. calcium

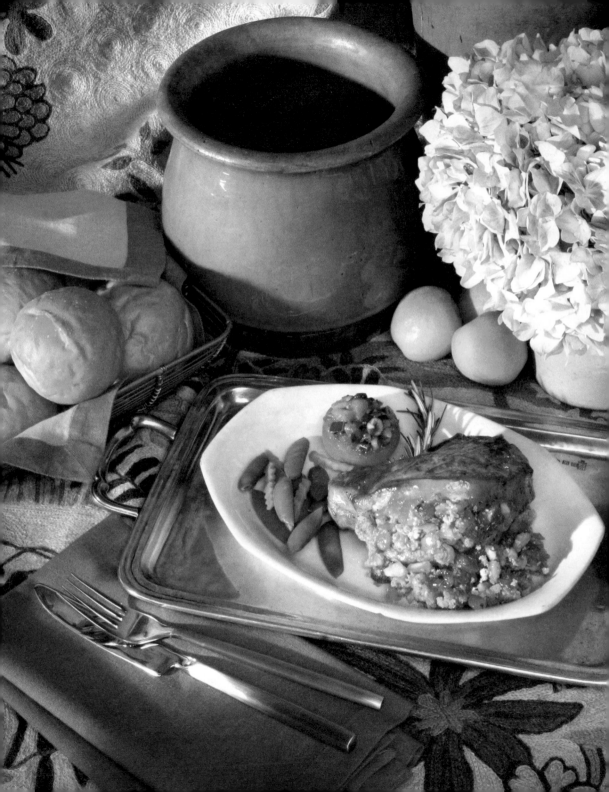

Apple & Apricot Stuffed Pork Chops

Thanks to Matt Rader
Associate Brand Director, Schick Intuition

This is a great-tasting and healthy way to spice up a classic pork chop, and is always a crowd pleaser. **The good news is**…it only looks difficult! Choose pork chops that are lean, or trim any fat before cooking.

INGREDIENTS

6	center cut pork chops, 1 inch thick
½ cup	chopped onion
½ cup	chopped celery
1 Tbsp.	olive oil
¼ cup each	soft bread crumbs, instant oats
½ cup	chopped apple (skin on or peeled, whichever you prefer)
⅓ cup	golden or dark raisins
1 Tbsp.	brown sugar
½ tsp.	ginger
¼ cup	apricot preserves, sugar free

PREPARATION

- Preheat oven to 325 degrees.
- Cut deep horizontal pocket in each chop.
- In medium skillet, cook onion and celery in oil until crisp and tender.
- Add bread crumbs, oats, apple, raisins, brown sugar, ginger and 2 Tbsp. of the preserves; mix well.
- Stuff each pork chop with about ¼ cup stuffing mixture.
- Place in ungreased 13″ x 9″ baking dish; cover.
- Bake at 325 degrees for 45 minutes.
- Uncover; spread top of chops with remaining 2 Tbsp. preserves.
- Bake uncovered an additional 15-20 minutes or until pork chops are tender.

NUTRITIONAL ANALYSIS
Serves: 6
Each serving contains:
178 calories
19 g. protein
9 g. carbohydrates
5 g. fat (2 g. saturated fat)
25 mg. calcium

Chapter 9
Aging Gracefully

"How old would you be if you didn't know
how old you were?"

— Florence Henderson,
after Satchel Paige

A simple pledge...

for aging gracefully begins with exercising your brain just as you exercise your body. Yes, we really have some brain exercises...and, they're fun!

So much has been written on the subject of aging that it seems by now there would be a handbook on how to do it with success. The truth is...aging is not something to be achieved; it is just a normal part of life to be enjoyed. Successful aging may simply be the ability to lead an active, productive life while growing older and to maintain independence and joy for life and all it has to offer.

By the year 2020, one in six Americans will be older than 65. The impact on almost every aspect of our culture and society by this massive and rapidly expanding segment of the population will be profoundly far-reaching in a variety of social, economic and health care areas. All of us will be affected in some way or another.

Although the physical aging of our bodies is unavoidable, people age at widely different rates. Genetics – what you inherit from your parents and other ancestors – has a major influence on how you age, along with environmental factors and lifestyle. For example, if your parents both lived into their 90s, and if you get plenty of exercise, practice good nutrition and handle stress effectively, statistically you'll probably live longer and better. Take advantage of the building blocks for healthy living and **TAKE A PLEDGE FOR BETTER HEALTH** today.

If you've made some simple pledges for nutrition and exercise found in Chapters 1 & 2, and you adhere to the building blocks for beauty found in Chapter 7...then you're off to a good start.

Simple Pledges...
for Graceful Aging

I pledge to: ☑

☐ Develop and maintain a strong social support network of family, friends and colleagues.

☐ Develop a personal exercise program combining aerobic, flexibility and weight-bearing activities.

☐ Take charge of my brain. Make an active commitment to learning and personal growth. I know that according to research on lifespan development, if I continue to use my brain and develop my intellect and if I remain socially connected and active, I can actually increase my IQ scores as I age.

☐ Take charge of my financial future. (NOTE: If you are single, don't count on getting married to finance your old age. If you are married, learn what is going on with your finances. If you are female, statistics say you will spend seven to 15 years or more as a widow, depending upon the age difference between you and your husband. You will probably be on your own for a long time. Plan, plan, plan.)

☐ Eat a low-fat, high-fiber diet complete with fruits, vegetables, grains, and legumes as much as possible. (See Chapter 1 for more information on nutrition.)

☐ Remain goal oriented. Regardless of my age, still set one, five, ten and 20-year goals.

☐ Remain active! I might get a part-time job, volunteer, spend time with children or animals, create hobbies, read books, go back to school, write a book or keep a journal to share my wisdom with others.

TAKE A PLEDGE FOR BETTER HEALTH at www.speakingofwomenshealth.com

Seeing The Future Clearly

Various malfunctions in the process of vision may occur as a person ages. They may be caused by reduced muscle tone and decreased eye lubrication. In addition, vision problems may result when various structures in the eye deteriorate or become diseased. The pupil gets smaller – as much as a third of its size by age 60 according to one estimate – altering how (and how much) light passes through it.

Here are the eye disorders and diseases that most commonly occur with age:

Age-related macular degeneration. This disease is the leading cause of blindness in people older than 50.

Glaucoma. Glaucoma is a leading cause of blindness in the United States.

Cataracts. The normally clear lens of the eye becomes progressively clouded, ultimately blocking light from reaching the retina or scattering light and creating glare.

Presbyopia. Almost everyone will develop this condition, typically starting around age 40. In presbyopia, the normally flexible lens of the eye becomes increasingly rigid and unable to focus on objects close-up.

To reduce your chances of developing any of these problems at a younger age, it is important that you have regular eye examinations beginning at age 40.

Senior Moments

Many older people worry about becoming more forgetful. They think forgetfulness is the first sign of Alzheimer's disease. In the past, memory loss and confusion were considered a normal part of aging. However, scientists now know that most people remain both alert and able as they age, although it may take them longer to remember things.

A lot of people experience memory lapses. Some memory problems are serious, and others are not. People who have serious changes in their memory, personality and behavior may suffer from a form of brain disease called dementia. Dementia seriously affects a person's ability to carry out daily activities. Alzheimer's disease is one of many types of dementia.

Building Blocks...
to Keep Your Brain Sharp!

What can you do today to keep your mind sharp? While many of us chuckle when we hear about those so-called "senior moments", those times we can't find our keys, can't remember someone's name, or forget why we came into a room once we get there. While we may believe this is just part of aging, many older adults may worry it's more than that. **The good news is**, that while many may fear Alzheimer's disease, only about 1 in 10 adults over the age 65 are affected.

What happens is that, just like our muscles, our brains get a little flabby without exercise. Dr. Larry Katz, researcher at Duke University Medical Center, and author of *Keep Your Brain Alive*, suggests these "fun exercises" to keep your brain fit. Here are some examples from his book:

- Turn the family pictures on your desk and night table upside down. This may confuse others but let them laugh.
- If you normally wear your watch on your left arm, wear it on your right.
- When you unlock your door, instead of looking for the keyhole, close your eyes and feel where it is.
- If you're right handed…try brushing your teeth with your left hand.

All of these tricks help to rebuild synapses or connectors in your brain. What's happening is, by breaking your routine you're forcing your brain to learn something new…this is why children learn so fast. Every day they build new connectors while learning new things for the first time…and, according to Dr. Katz, those synapses are also pathways for memory.

So, to keep your memory in tip-top shape, exercise it!

The term dementia describes a group of symptoms that are caused by changes in brain function. Dementia symptoms may include asking the same questions repeatedly; becoming lost in familiar places; being unable to follow directions; getting disoriented about time, people, and places; and neglecting personal safety, hygiene, and nutrition. People with dementia lose their abilities at different rates. Dementia is caused by many conditions. Some conditions that cause dementia can be reversed, and others cannot. Sometimes emotional problems may lead to confusion, forgetfulness and other symptoms of dementia. With professional treatment and doctor's care, these are reversible.

Symptoms Of Alzheimer's Disease

Symptoms begin slowly and become steadily worse. As the disease progresses, symptoms range from mild forgetfulness to serious impairments in thinking, judgement, and the ability to perform daily activities. Eventually, patients may need total care.

For some people in the early and middle stages of Alzheimer's disease, new medications have been developed to possibly delay the worsening of some of the disease's symptoms. For some, doctors may prescribe medications to reduce agitation, anxiety, depression or sleeping problems – all symptoms of Alzheimer's disease.

Family members and friends can assist people with dementia in continuing their daily routines, physical activities, and social contacts. People with dementia should be kept up-to-date about the details of their lives, such as the time of day, where they live, and what is happening at home or in the world.

The most common form of dementia in older people is Alzheimer's disease. In Alzheimer's disease, nerve cell changes in certain parts of the brain result in the death of a large number of cells.

As you age, your body secretes smaller amounts of key chemicals that help your body decide when to sleep and when to wake up. Levels of growth hormone, which promote deep sleep, and melatonin, which regulates your sleeping and waking cycle, decrease as you age.

Get Your ZZZZZZZs

Many older adults struggle with getting a good night's sleep. Like food and water, adequate sleep is essential for good health and quality of life. Not sleeping well can lead to a number of problems. For example, older adults who have poor nighttime sleep are more likely to have a depressed mood, attention and memory problems, excessive daytime sleepiness, more nighttime falls, and may use more over-the-counter or prescription sleep aids. Sleep problems also are associated with a poor quality of life.

Here are some tips for a good night's sleep, from the National Institutes of Health.

✔ Follow a regular schedule – go to sleep and wake up at the same time, even on weekends. Sticking to a regular bedtime and wake time schedule helps keep you in sync with your body's circadian clock, a 24-hour internal rhythm affected by sunlight.

✔ Try not to nap too much during the day – you might be less sleepy at night.

✔ Try to exercise at regular times each day. Exercising regularly improves the quality of your nighttime sleep and helps you sleep more soundly. Try to finish your workout at least three hours before bedtime.

✔ Try to get some natural light in the afternoon each day.

✔ Be careful about what you eat. Don't drink beverages with caffeine late in the day. Caffeine is a stimulant and can keep you awake. Also, if you like a snack before bed, a warm beverage and a few crackers may help.

✔ Don't drink alcohol or smoke cigarettes to help you sleep. Even small amounts of alcohol can make it harder to stay asleep. Smoking is dangerous for many reasons, including the hazard of falling asleep with a lit cigarette. Also, the nicotine in cigarettes is a stimulant.

✔ Create a safe and comfortable place to sleep. Make sure there are locks on all doors and smoke alarms on each floor. A lamp that's easy to turn on and a phone by your bed may be helpful. The room should be dark, well ventilated, and as quiet as possible.

✔ Develop a bedtime routine. Do the same things each night to tell your body that it's time to wind down. Some people watch the evening news, read a book or soak in a warm bath.

✔ Use your bedroom only for sleeping. After turning off the light, give yourself about 15 minutes to fall asleep. If you are still awake and not drowsy, get out of bed. When you get sleepy, go back to bed.

✔ Try not to worry about your sleep. Some people find that playing mental games is helpful. For example, think black – a black cat on a black velvet pillow on a black corduroy sofa, etc. Or, tell yourself it's five minutes before you have to get up and you're just trying to get a few extra winks.

Trouble sleeping? Talk to your pharmacist about medications you're taking and the chance that they might be causing your sleepless nights. If that's the case, talk to your doctor about changing the time of day you take your medication.

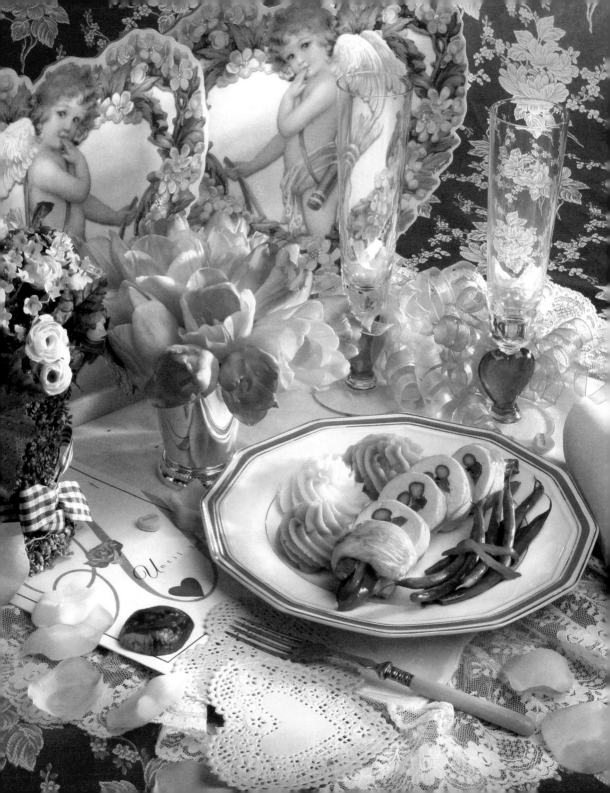

Rolled Chicken

Thanks to Valerie Simpson, Singer & Songwriter
Spokesperson, National Minority Health Initiative

Valerie tells us this is a favorite of hers that she first tried at our National Speaking of Women's Health Sponsor Recognition Dinner. We think you'll agree!

INGREDIENTS

- 4 chicken breasts, boneless & skinless
- 4 sprigs of rosemary
  cooking spray
- ¼ cup flour (all purpose)
- 8 stalks of asparagus, trimmed to 3″ in length
- 1 red bell pepper, cored and cut into strips
  salt & pepper to taste

PREPARATION

- Place chicken, boned side up, on cutting board. Working from center out, pound chicken lightly with wooden mallet to make cutlets about ¼ inch thick.
- Sprinkle with salt & pepper.
- Place a rosemary sprig, 2 stalks of asparagus, and 2 strips of red pepper in center of each cutlet.
- Tuck in sides of each, and roll up (like a jelly roll), pressing to seal well. Skewer or tie securely.
- Coat rolls in flour. Brown lightly in olive oil and remove from skillet, transferring to baking dish, lightly coated with cooking spray.
- Bake at 350 degrees for 35 minutes.
- Remove from oven. Cut each "roll" into slices. Serve.

NUTRITIONAL ANALYSIS
Serves: 4
Each serving (4 oz. chicken) contains approximately:
269 calories
36 g. protein
17 g. carbohydrates
12 g. fat (4 g. saturated fat)
70 mg. calcium

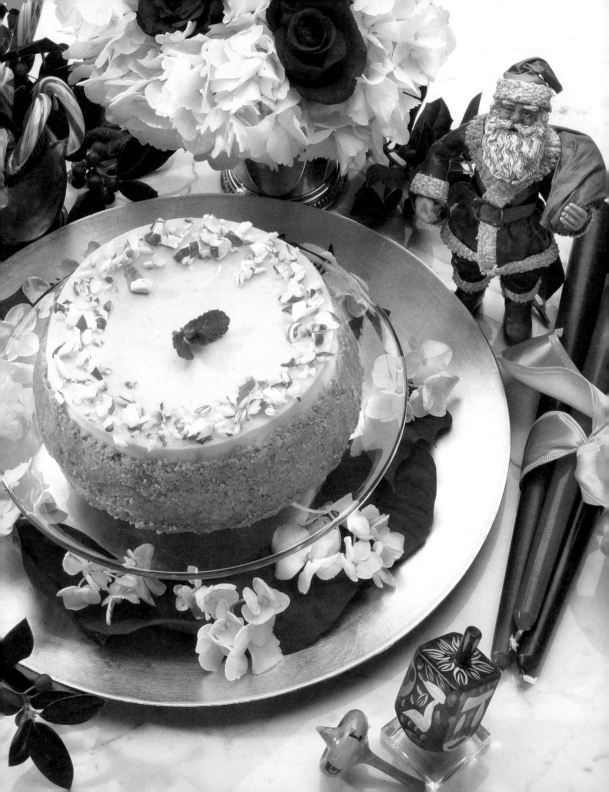

Peppermint Patty Cheesecake

Thanks to Carol Hamilton
President & General Manager, L'Oreal Paris

Put those candy canes to extra use with this scrumptious dessert from Canyon Ranch. Serving–sized pieces can be individually wrapped and kept frozen to give as gifts. Enjoy!

INGREDIENTS

Crust
¾ cup	graham cracker crumbs, regular or chocolate (4½ whole crackers)
1 Tbsp.	water

Filling
3 cups	fat-free cream cheese (24 oz.), at room temperature
1	egg
4	egg whites
¾ cup	plus 2 Tbsp. fat-free sweetened condensed skim milk
¼ cup	all-purpose flour
2 Tbsp.	fructose
1 tsp.	peppermint extract
3	small peppermint candies (candy canes) coarsely chopped

PREPARATION

- Preheat the oven to 300 degrees.
- Spray a 9″ springform cake pan with non-stick cooking spray.
- Combine the graham cracker crumbs and water in a bowl. Mix until moistened. Press into the bottom of the pan.
- Combine all remaining ingredients, except the peppermint candies, in a bowl. Beat with electric mixer until smooth.
- Spoon the batter into the pan on top of the crust. Sprinkle the candies around the top edge of the cheesecake.
- Bake in preheated oven for 35–40 minutes, until cake is firm but, the center moves slightly when touched.
- Cool completely on a wire rack. Refrigerate, tightly covered, for at least 4 hours, or overnight before serving.

NUTRITIONAL ANALYSIS
Servings: 16
Each serving contains approximately:
135 calories
4 g. protein
19 g. carbohydrates
2 g. fat
38 mg. calcium

Chapter 10
Personal and Family Safety

"It takes a village to raise a child."

— African Proverb

A simple pledge...

for personal and family safety begins with learning what to do to treat your family's bumps and bruises to something as serious as CPR. *Even something as simple as pledging to have a first-aid kit, and knowing what's inside it, can give you the confidence for the next building blocks of sports safety, swimming pool accidents and home preparedness. Your first simple pledge may even be as easy as not being afraid to call 9-1-1.*

As women, we are called upon to take care of many people – our children, husbands, friends, parents, neighbors, aging relatives, and, ourselves. Often our homes are filled with people…our own kids, their friends, the neighbors' kids. When children or family members become sick or injured, Mom is often the first to be consulted. This chapter will discuss personal and family safety and arm you with the two most vital ingredients for safety….education and preparedness!

First, Be Prepared!

Arm yourself with proper medicines and products to treat common injuries, ailments and illness. A well-stocked medicine cabinet is a good start.

According to the American Red Cross, a well-stocked cabinet should include:

- ✔ Adhesive bandages
- ✔ Adhesive tape
- ✔ Alcohol wipes
- ✔ Analgesic (relieves pain)
- ✔ Antacid (relieves upset stomach)
- ✔ Antibiotic ointment (reduces risk of infection)
- ✔ Antihistamine (relieves allergy symptoms)
- ✔ Mentholated chest rub
- ✔ Antiseptic (helps stop infection)
- ✔ Calibrated measuring spoon
- ✔ Disposable hot wrap and refreezable ice pack
- ✔ Decongestant (relieves stuffy nose and other cold symptoms)
- ✔ Disinfectant

- ✔ Fever reducer (adult and child). Do not give aspirin to children. Check with your pharmacist for a suitable substitute for reducing a child's fever.
- ✔ Gauze pads
- ✔ Hydrocortisone (relieves itching and inflammation)
- ✔ Syrup of ipecac (induces vomiting) and activated charcoal (absorbs poison, use when syrup of ipecac isn't recommended). Give syrup of ipecac or activated charcoal only after talking with your doctor or a Poison Control Center expert. Some ingested poisons are treated differently. *If you have a poisoning emergency, call 1-800-222-1222.*
- ✔ Thermometer
- ✔ Tweezers

First Aid Kits

Be prepared away from home by keeping a first aid kit on hand in the car, boat, barn, backpack or other place. You can purchase kits, or assemble one yourself. Some kits are specifically created for particular activities like boating, hiking, etc.

Medicine Safety

According to Wal-Mart pharmacist Karen Froendhoff, some simple precautions will protect your family when taking medications.

✔ Remember that even over-the-counter medications and vitamins can cause serious problems, and even death, if a child or elderly person is overdosed.

✔ Only give family members medicines that have been prescribed specifically for them.

✔ Use the correct dose and read the label carefully.

✔ Follow the directions carefully, and do not confuse teaspoon (tsp.) with tablespoon (Tbsp.). If the medicine came with a measuring device, such as a dropper, medicine cup or dosing spoon, only use it and do not substitute another device when administering it to your child. A kitchen teaspoon is not appropriate for use in measuring medication.

✔ If a family member is already taking a medication, make sure that any other new medicines are compatible before combining.

✔ Consult your pharmacist about combining prescription medications with over-the-counter drugs, including vitamins and herbal supplements.

Inventory your medicine cabinet and first aid kits at least once a year:

✔ Check expiration dates. Throw out all outdated medicine. If you're not sure about a certain item, call your pharmacist and ask what the shelf life of the medicine is.

✔ If medications are not in original containers or labeled clearly, throw them away. It's dangerous to store medicines in anything but their original containers. Some medicines come in tinted glass, for example, because exposure to light may cause deterioration.

✔ Every medication is a potential poison. If there are children in the house, keep all medicines and vitamins locked in a high cabinet, well out of reach.

Simple Pledges...
for Home Safety

I pledge to: ✔

☐ Equip my home with smoke and fire detectors, as well as a fire extinguisher in the kitchen, garage, workshop or other areas where fire may occur. I will check batteries in each detector twice a year. (NOTE: Be certain your home is free of carbon monoxide gases. At-home detectors are available.)

☐ Childproof my home, even if children are there just occasionally. This includes safety latches on cabinets and doors, closed doors near stairwells, childproof caps or a locked cabinet for medications, locked poisons and household detergents and child safety barriers for electrical outlets.

☐ Be sure all guns and firearms in my home or garage, are stored in a locked cabinet. I will store bullets in a separate locked location and talk to my children about gun safety at home and in others' homes.

☐ Teach my children to practice safe habits around animals, even if they belong to someone they know. Animals can be unpredictable. I will tell them to always ask permission from the owner before approaching an animal.

☐ Learn CPR and basic first aid, and require that regular babysitters take a basic first aid class.

☐ Teach my children to call 9-1-1 in the event of an emergency. (Even very young children can save lives.)

TAKE A PLEDGE FOR BETTER HEALTH at www.speakingofwomenshealth.com

Safety At Home

According to the American Red Cross, fires are among the deadliest disasters to destroy homes across the country. Each year, nearly 5,000 Americans die in fires, and 80% of those deaths occur in home fires. Most residential fires are preventable.

Preparedness is your best weapon against deadly fires. Follow these simple steps to make your home "fire safe".

✔ Determine at least two ways to escape from every room of your home. Consider escape ladders for sleeping areas on the second or third floors. Learn how to use them and store them near the windows.

✔ Select a location outside your home where everyone would meet after escaping.

✔ Practice your escape plan at least twice a year by holding family fire drills. Experts know that even young children can save lives. Be certain your children understand the dangers of fire and how to get out of the home should one occur.

✔ When staying in hotels, make a game out of seeing who can locate the nearest fire exits when you arrive.

Consider a family outing unlike others...take a first aid course together! Learn the basics of minor emergency care, accident prevention, CPR and AED (automated external defibrillator) use. Your local Red Cross or other organization is a great resource for safety courses. Consider inviting your neighbors, church family, or even the parents from the soccer team to join you!

Building Blocks...
for Surviving Emergencies

A Prescription for Safety...Don't Leave Home Without It!

The most important item to have in the event of a medical emergency is information. In the event of an emergency, when your emotions are at their peak, written and accurate information may save a life. Include:

- Allergies. List any medication, food or latex allergies or sensitivities your family member may have.

- An updated list of your family's medications, including dosage.

- Any pre-existing illness or surgeries. Don't leave anything out. If a family member has a chronic condition such as diabetes, asthma or is allergic to medications, doctors suggest that they wear an identifying alert bracelet or necklace.

In the event of an asthma attack, the victim should not be left alone until the attack has subsided after proper use of inhaled medications. If the inhaler is not readily available, accompany the victim to the location of the inhaler. Each moment is precious.

Follow these safety tips in the event that a fire strikes.

✔ Once you are out, stay out! Call the fire department from a neighbor's home.

✔ If you see smoke or fire in your first escape route, use your second way out. If you must exit through smoke, crawl low under the smoke to your exit. If you are escaping through a closed door, feel the door before opening it. If it is warm, use your second way out.

✔ If smoke, heat or flames block your exit routes, stay in the room with the door closed. Signal for help using a bright-colored cloth at the window. If there is a telephone in the room, call the fire department and tell them where you are.

Travel Safety

Whether your plans call for a week-long trip or just a day-trip by car, it pays to keep some simple safety tips in mind.

Traveling by car?

✔ Make sure your car is road-worthy before you start. Check oil level, the transmission fluid, the radiator's anti-freeze/coolant level, the windshield washer fluid, the brake fluid, the battery and all the cables.

✔ Remember to drive defensively and safely.

✔ Plan your route in advance and have a good map on hand.

✔ Keep your doors and trunk locked to protect your valuables.

✔ Always follow safety rules: use your seat belt, be sure children are properly secured in car seats, and always have a designated driver.

Use Your Head! Be Sure There's A Helmet On It!

BE CERTAIN THAT YOUR CHILDREN WEAR A HELMET WHEN ON WHEELS, *whether it's bikes, blades or skateboards! And, while you're at it...the best way to teach is by example. Make this a family rule!*

Once you arrive...

✔ Remain alert and aware of your surroundings at all times.

✔ Make note of exits and exit routes whenever you enter new places (hotels, restaurants, shopping malls, theaters, concert halls, etc.).

✔ Consider leaving expensive jewelry at home, or in the hotel's safe.

✔ Consider travel insurance.

Rx for safe travels

✔ If you are flying, keep your medications in your carry-on luggage so that you have access to them during your flight and will not lose them in the event that your luggage gets lost. Plus, keeping your medications with you helps prevent exposure to extreme temperatures in the baggage compartment, which may alter the drug's effectiveness. Keep in mind, airport security requires that your medications be in their original, labeled containers.

✔ If your medication requires you to use a syringe (insulin, for instance) you may need to carry your prescription with you to ensure that you can pass through airport security.

✔ If you are traveling through several time zones, ask your pharmacist to work out a specific plan for adjusting the timing and dosage of your medications. This will prevent you from taking too much or too little.

✔ If you are visiting a hot, humid climate, be sure to keep your medications in a cool, dry place out of direct sunlight. Never store medications in the glove compartment of your car.

✔ Take along more medication than the number of days you've planned to be away. This will allow you to be prepared for unexpected delays.

First Aid Basics

If the last time you learned basic first aid was in grade school or high school, much of the information has not changed, but much is new, too.

The rise in the spread of blood borne disease, including AIDS and hepatitis, has led to a whole new emphasis on protecting one's self from exposure to another person's blood or body fluids. Although the risk of contracting a disease is rare, according to the American Red Cross, the following precautions can reduce your risk:

1. Avoid contact with blood and other body fluids.

2. Use protective equipment, such as disposable gloves (available at any drug store) and breathing masks.

3. Thoroughly wash your hands with soap and water immediately after giving care to someone else.

If you do have to clean up a blood spill, do so immediately or as soon as possible after it occurs. Use disposable gloves and a breathing barrier, and wipe up the spill with paper towels or other absorbent material. Then flood the area with a solution of water and bleach (one gallon of water, ¼ cup bleach), allow it to stand for 20 minutes and then wipe it carefully. Throw away all material used in the cleanup in a labeled biohazard container.

Treating Shock: ABCs

No matter what the injury, someone administering first aid should always be on the lookout for shock. Shock means that the body has suffered a tremendous injury or trauma of some kind. Shock can be brought on by a severe injury, loss of blood, a life-threatening allergic reaction, poisoning or other event.

When shock occurs, the body's blood pressure drops suddenly, and the heart is not able to provide enough blood to the body's tissues. Signs of shock include:

✔ Restlessness or irritability

✔ Nausea and vomiting

✔ An altered level of consciousness (confused or dazed)

✔ Pale or ashen skin; cool or moist skin

✔ A blue tinge to the lips and fingernails

✔ Rapid or shallow breathing

✔ Rapid heartbeat

What to do if you suspect shock:

✔ Call 9-1-1

✔ Monitor the victim's **ABCs** – **A**irway, **B**reathing and **C**irculation

✔ Control any external bleeding

✔ Keep the victim from getting chilled or overheated

✔ Elevate the victim's legs about 12 inches – but only if you do not suspect a head, neck or back injury or do not suspect broken bones in the hips or legs.

WARNING – *If there is any chance of trauma or severe injury to the head, neck or spinal cord, never, ever attempt to move the victim. Moving the victim could further damage the spinal cord causing permanent paralysis or brain injury. The only exception to this rule is if the victim is under water. In this instance, bring the victim to the surface to enable breathing, taking care to support the head and neck as much as possible.*

✔ Comfort and reassure the victim until advanced medical personnel arrive and take over. Do not give food or drink to someone in shock.

Controlling Bleeding

If someone is bleeding, follow these steps:

✔ Put on disposable gloves to protect yourself.

✔ Cover the wound with a dressing (gauze, clean cloth) and press firmly and directly against the wound.

✔ Elevate the injured area so that it is held above the victim's heart – but do this ONLY when you suspect that a bone is not broken.

✔ Cover the wound by rolling it in gauze or a dressing, tear small strips at the end and tie a knot directly over the wound.

✔ If the bleeding does not stop, apply additional dressing and bandages. Apply pressure directly to the wound to squeeze the artery against the bone and call 9-1-1 or have someone near you call 9-1-1. Look for signs of shock.

Special Injury Situations

Eye injuries: If someone injures the eye or has an object embedded in the eye, do not attempt to remove the object. Place the victim in a comfortable position and place a sterile dressing around the eye and the object, stabilizing it as best you can. Apply a bandage but do not put direct pressure on the eyeball. Seek medical treatment as soon as possible.

Chemicals in the eye: Quick treatment is required if chemicals or other dangerous substances get into the eye, because blindness or permanent damage can occur quickly. Symptoms of eye contamination include extreme pain, and the victim may or not be able to open the affected eye. Usually, the eye will water a lot, become red and swell.

Suggestions for treatment include:

✔ Do not touch the victim's eye, and don't let the victim touch it, either. Put on protective gloves, if possible.

✔ Hold the victim's head under a water faucet so that water runs over the eye for at least 10 minutes. Make sure the water that rinses away from the eye does not splash you or the victim, because it can be contaminated, too. If a faucet is not available or does not accommodate someone's head underneath it, use a pitcher or glass to pour the water.

✔ If the victim cannot open the eye, gently pull apart the eyelids to clean all parts of the eye and eyelids.

✔ Place a sterile pad or clean pad made of non-fluff materials over the eye, and ask the victim to hold it in place. If possible, identify the chemical or substance that caused the problem, and make sure the victim is treated in an emergency room.

Nosebleed: Lean the victim forward (Yes, forward!) and pinch the nostrils together until bleeding stops.

Tooth knocked out: Place a sterile dressing directly in the space left by the tooth and ask the victim to bite down gently to apply direct pressure. Preserve the tooth by placing it in a container of cool, fresh milk or water. Always try to handle the tooth by the chewing edge, not the root. Get the victim and the tooth to a dentist immediately. The sooner the victim is treated, the better the chance of saving and re-implanting the tooth.

CPR – Cardiopulmonary Resuscitation

CPR is a form of intervention, usually administered to someone whose heart has stopped beating and who is no longer breathing. If only the breathing has stopped, rescue breathing alone can be administered to keep air flowing in and out of the lungs.

CPR is a two-stage approach in which the person providing first aid keeps pumping the victim's heart to keep blood flowing and blows air into the lungs to keep oxygen circulating through the body. It's always done until professional emergency medical help arrives.

First, Call 9-1-1 For Emergency Help.

To administer CPR:

First, lay the victim on his/her back. Find the correct position for your hands on the victim's chest. Using your hand that's closest to the victim's feet, use two fingers to locate the notch on the lower end of the victim's sternum (the breastbone, or bottom of the rib cage). Slide your middle and index fingers up to the edge of the rib cage to that notch where the ribs meet the breastbone. Place your middle finger in the notch, your index finger above it, and the heel of your other hand just above your index finger on the breastbone. This is the area of the chest where you must apply downward pressure. Now place the heel of your first hand on top of the other hand, interlocking the fingers so that the fingers of bottom hand are raised off the victim's chest.

1. Give 15 compressions, or downward thrusts. Position your shoulders over your hands and compress the chest – pushing downward – about two inches. Do 15 compressions in about 10 seconds, and keep the up-and-down movements smooth. Keep your hand in contact with the victim's chest at all times.

2. Now shift to the person's head and mouth to give rescue breaths. Open the person's airway by tilting the head backwards and lifting the chin. Pinch the victim's nose shut and seal your lips tightly around the person's mouth. Give two rescue breaths into the person's mouth, each lasting about 2 seconds. Watch the victim's chest rise to be sure your breaths go in.

3. Repeat the compression/breathing cycles – 3 more sets of 15 compressions and 2 more breathing rescue sessions.

4. After one minute, check the person's circulation for no more than 10 seconds…look, listen and feel for breathing.

5. If the person has a pulse and is breathing, keep the airway open, monitor the breathing and wait for emergency help to arrive.

6. If the person has a pulse but still is not breathing, continue to do rescue breathing and check the circulation signs about every minute. Wait for medical help to arrive.

7. If the person has no pulse and is not breathing, continue administering CPR – 15 compressions followed by 2 rescue breaths – until help arrives, checking the person's pulse every few minutes.

Why Is It Important To Perform Rescue Breathing?

When the body is deprived of oxygen, the brain begins to die within 4-6 minutes. Rescue breathing is a way of keeping oxygen flowing into the person's lungs and throughout the bloodstream if the victim is unconscious or is having a breathing emergency – an asthma attack, for example, or is in shock. And when it comes to rescue breathing, time is of the essence.

In Conclusion...

As you have read this book, we hope you have learned lots of new information and reinforced what you already know. At Speaking of Women's Health, our mission is "to educate women to make informed decisions about their health, well-being and personal safety". Join us this year to **TAKE A PLEDGE FOR BETTER HEALTH**, because small changes really do make a difference. We hope you will be an important part of this grass roots movement. Taking this pledge online at **www.speakingofwomenshealth.com** can be your first Building Block toward a healthier, happier life for you and your family.

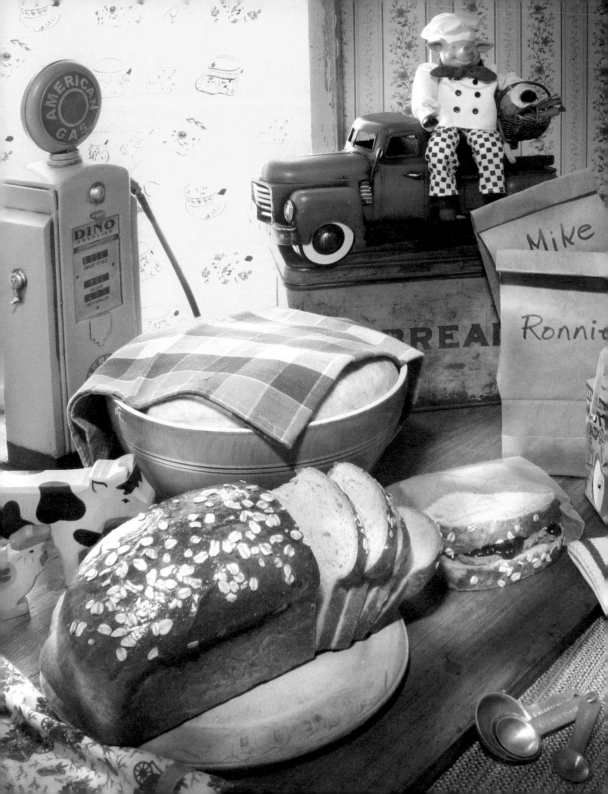

Oats & Honey Bread

Thanks to Karen Stuckey
Sr. Vice President, General Merchandising Manager
Products & Trend Development, Wal-Mart

Whether you prefer to knead and bake in a loaf or want to use your bread machine, this bread recipe will be a favorite. The rich oats are healthy and add texture, and the slight honey-sweet taste is sure to please!

INGREDIENTS

2 tsp.	olive oil
1¾ cups	warm water (105°F to 110°F)
1 Tbsp.	dry yeast
¾ cup	quick-cooking oats & additional for garnish
⅓ cup	honey
3 Tbsp.	vegetable oil
2½ tsp.	salt
(about) 5 cups	all purpose flour OR try a 50/50 white & wheat blend for added flavor
1 large	egg, slightly beaten

PREPARATION

- Stir ¼ cup warm water and yeast in large bowl. Let stand 10 minutes to dissolve yeast.
- Stir in remaining 1½ cups water, ¾ cup oats, honey, oil and salt.
- Stir in enough flour to form soft dough.
- Coat another large bowl with oil. Transfer dough to oiled bowl and turn to coat.
- Cover with plastic wrap (spray with cooking spray first to keep it from sticking to dough), then kitchen towel and let rise at room temperature until doubled in volume, about 1 hour.
- Oil two 8½" x 4½" x 2½" loaf pans.
- Punch down dough; shape into 2 loaves. Place 1 loaf in each pan.
- Cover and let rise in warm draft-free area until almost doubled in volume, about 20 minutes.
- Preheat oven to 350 degrees F.
- Brush tops of loaves with egg; sprinkle with additional oats for garnish.
- Bake until brown on top and tester inserted into center comes out clean, about 40 minutes.
- Cool completely.

NUTRITIONAL ANALYSIS
Yield: 2 small loaves
Two slices contain approximately:
102 calories
1 g. protein
12 g. carbohydrates
6 g. fat (1 g. saturated fat)
6 mg. calcium

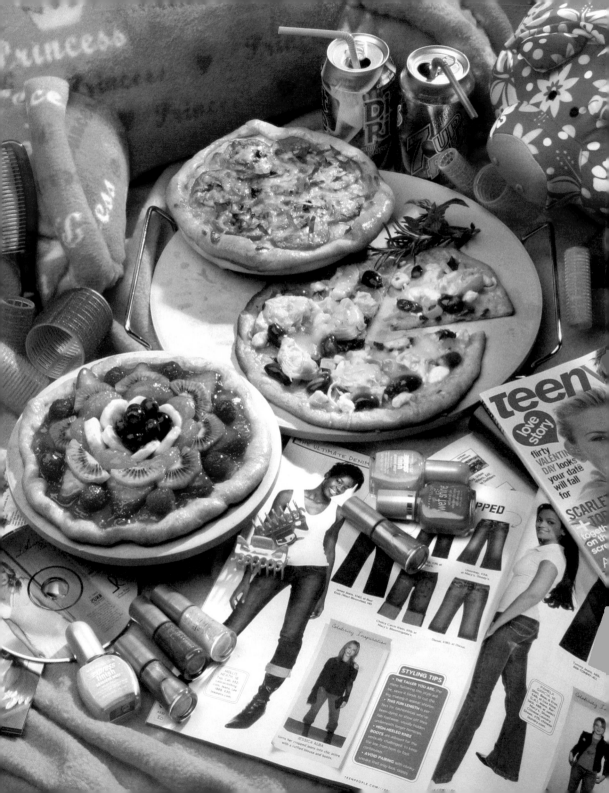

Party Pizzas

Ellen Bowman, PhD
Director, Global Health Care External Relations, P&G

Everyone loves a great pizza, and contrary to what many believe, pizza can be both nutritious and delicious! Experiment with different toppings – brush olive oil on the crust and then add artichoke hearts, herbs, olives, sun-dried tomatoes, spinach leaves…or, serve this dessert pizza and the whole family will love it! Who needs to know it's healthy?!

INGREDIENTS

1 pkg. refrigerated pizza dough

¼ cup sugar-free preserves (choose your favorite flavor, we used blackberry)

Fresh fruits, sliced
  strawberries
  kiwifruit
  mandarin oranges
  (canned and drained)
  raspberries
  blueberries
  blackberries
  bananas

PREPARATION

- Prepare crust as directed on package. Bake and let cool.
- Spread preserves to edge of partially-cooled dough.
- Beginning at the edge, arrange fruit in rows, working your way inside in a spiral.
- Serve chilled. Enjoy!

NUTRITIONAL ANALYSIS - Pizza crust, prepared
Servings per recipe: 6
Each slice contains approximately:
160 calories
5 g. protein
31 g. carbohydrates
2 g. fat (0 saturated fat)

Index

Aerobic Activity 21
Allergies (food) 130
Alzheimer's Disease 115-117
Anthocyanins 41
Antioxidants 11, 34
Beta-Carotene 53
Biotin...40
Bisphosphonate 51
Blood Pressure 9, 20, 35-37, 40, 101, 133
Bone(s) 19-24, 47-53, 71, 134
Bone Density 19, 48, 51-52
Bra(s) 22
Breast 22, 33, 71-73
Breathing 8, 23, 39, 61, 133-137
Caffeine........................62, 73, 76, 102, 118
Calcium 11, 48, 49, 51-53, 62, 93, 104
Cancer............5, 33, 37, 48, 85, 86, 88, 106
Carbohydrates 8-10, 40-41,
    52, 73, 103
Cardiovascular Diseases 33
Chocolate 77, 103
Cholesterol....................................11, 33-37
Colon Cancer 106
Constipation 76, 104-105
C-Reactive Protein (CRP) 37
Dairy Products...............................8, 48, 53
Dehydration................................23, 73
Dementia..115, 117
Depression 62, 70-72, 117
DEXA 48
Diabetes 35-37, 41, 101, 130
Esophagus.......................................100-103
Estrogen 48, 52, 70-75
Exercise ..4, 8, 19-25, 33, 47-50, 53, 60, 63,
    71, 73, 74, 90, 104, 113-118
Fats..................................8, 10-11, 41
Fiber.................9, 11, 36, 41, 104-105, 114
Fish................8, 10, 13, 34, 40-41, 53
Flexibility 21, 53, 114

Folate 41
Friends, Friendships ..23, 59, 62, 69, 77, 93,
    114, 117, 125
Fruits 7-13, 33-34, 40-41, 49, 76, 84,
    87, 104, 107, 114
Gas...72, 103
Gastro Esophageal Reflux Disease
    (GERD) 11, 100-106
Hair 11, 68, 71, 83, 86, 89-93
Hair Color 86, 90
Hair Loss 91, 93
Heart Attack 32-38
Heart Disease 9, 11, 32-37, 40-41, 69-71,
    101, 105
Heartburn......................................99-107
Hydrogenated (Trans) Fats 8
Iron 11, 40, 89, 93, 104
Irritable Bowel Syndrome (IBS) 11, 100,
    105, 106
Keratin..93
Kegel Exercises 75
Lactose Intolerant 11
Legumes 13, 34, 40-41, 53, 114
Lycopene 41
Magnesium 11, 34, 41, 49, 52
Manganese..11, 53
Medication(s) 52, 91, 119, 127, 130, 132
Memory 20, 115, 116, 118
Menopause............34-35, 48, 51-52, 60, 69,
    71-75, 91, 104
Mental Health...63
Minerals...9, 52, 93
Moisturizer(s) 63, 84, 86
Nail(s) 93, 111
Niacin 40
Nutrition...................4, 7-13, 113-114, 117
Obesity 8, 37, 71
Omega-3 Fats 8, 34, 41
Omega-6 Fats...8

Osteoporosis............................19, 47-53, 74
Pantothenic Acid 40
Parathyroid Hormone (PTH) 52
Peri-menopause 72
Phosphorous 52
Phytochemicals 87
Phytoestrogens..53
Polyps...106
Portion (serving size) 8-13
Potassium 11, 34, 40-41
Pre-menstrual Syndrome (PMS)........62, 71
Progesterone 70, 72
Prostate 11
Protein 8, 11, 37, 49, 52, 89, 93
Recipes:
    Apple & Apricot Stuffed Pork Chops 111
    Awesome Smoothie 15
    Beef & Broccoli with Ginger 109
    Beef Stew 67
    Chalupa..97
    Chicken Soup 79
    Colorful Mashed Potatoes 65
    Delicious Crab Salad 17
    Egg White Omelet 27
    Grilled Kabobs 45
    Hummus 57
    Moroccan Couscous Steak Salad 55
    Oats & Honey Bread 139
    Party Pizzas 141
    Peppermint Patty Cheesecake 123
    Rolled Chicken...................................121
    Salmon Salad 43
    Traditional Gazpacho 95
    Vi's Sunday Greens..............................81
    White Bean Chili 29
Reflux 100-101
Relaxation 11, 22-23, 73, 90, 107
Screenings 48, 99
Shoes 22, 51

Skin ..10-11, 20, 22, 41, 61, 74, 82-93, 133
Sleep 20, 61-63, 84, 118-119
Smoking....34, 36, 53, 84, 90, 101-102, 119
Sodium 9, 11, 13, 52, 73
SPF (Sun Protection Factor)..19, 63, 84-85
SSRI (Selective Serotonin Reuptake
    Inhibitor)...72
Stress 19, 23, 33, 40, 60, 71, 73, 75,
    91, 100, 113
Stress Incontinence.................................75
Stretching 19, 21, 25, 53
Sudden Cardiac Arrest (SCA) 32, 39
Sunscreen..................19, 49, 63, 84-86, 88
Synapses...116
Testosterone 48, 70-71
Transient Ischemic Attack (TIA) 34
Triglyceride(s) 37
Vegetables.................7-11, 34, 40-41, 52-53,
    84, 87, 104, 114
Vessels 32
Vitamin A 53, 93
Vitamin B.............................52, 89-90, 93
Vitamin B$_6$ 40-41, 63
Vitamin B$_{12}$ 63
Vitamin C 34, 41, 93
Vitamin D 48-49, 53
Vitamin E 11, 41
Vitamin K 53
Vitamins ..9, 11, 49, 52, 63, 87-90, 93, 127
Walking 8, 20-25, 39, 47, 50-51, 53
Water...............11-12, 21, 23, 40, 73, 75-76,
    84, 90, 104-105, 118, 133-135
Weight 8, 19-24, 35, 37, 47, 50, 53,
    62, 70-72, 75, 102, 105-107
Weight-Bearing Exercises 20-24,
    47, 50, 53, 114
Yoga............20-21, 23-24, 50, 53, 61-62, 73
Yogurt 8-10, 12-13, 52-53, 87
Zinc 49, 53, 89, 93

Important Phone Numbers

EMERGENCY **9-1-1**

Poison Control Center **1-800-222-1222**

Police Department . . . . _____

Fire Department . . . . _____

Our Home Phone Number . . . . _____

Our Home Address: _____

_____

Dad's Work . . . . _____

Dad's Cell Phone . . . . _____

Mom's Work . . . . _____

Mom's Cell Phone . . . . _____

Neighbor's Name _____   Phone _____

Neighbor's Name _____   Phone _____

Nearest Relative _____   Phone _____

Hospital _____   Phone _____

Physician _____   Phone _____

Dentist _____   Phone _____

School _____   Phone _____

School _____   Phone _____

Other Important Numbers _____

_____

SPECIAL INSTRUCTIONS _____

_____

_____